THE NEW
FATHER'S
PANIC BOOK

THE NEW FATHER'S PANIC BOOK

EVERYTHING A DAD NEEDS TO KNOW TO WELCOME HIS BUNDLE OF JOY

GENE B. WILLIAMS

AVON BOOKS ◆ NEW YORK

AVON BOOKS, INC.
1350 Avenue of the Americas
New York, New York 10019

Copyright © 1997 by Gene B. Williams
Interior design by Kellan Peck
Published by arrangement with the author
Visit our website at **http://www.AvonBooks.com**
ISBN: 0-380-78906-X

Library of Congress Cataloging in Publication Data:

Williams, Gene B.
   The new father's panic book / Gene B. Williams.
      p.   cm.
1. Pregnancy—Popular works. 2. Childbirth—Popular works. 3. Fathers—Popular works. I. Title.
RG525.W633   1997   96-39433
618.2—dc21   CIP

First Avon Books Trade Paperback Printing: June 1997

AVON TRADEMARK REG. U.S. PAT. OFF. AND IN OTHER COUNTRIES, MARCA REGISTRADA, HECHO EN U.S.A.

Printed in the U.S.A.

OPM 10 9 8 7 6 5 4 3

To the hundreds of fathers and mothers
who contributed their stories, and their time,
with a special thanks to
the fathers and mothers who are "in the soup."
Mostly—to fathers everywhere!

Contents

THE NEW FATHER'S PANIC BOOK

Introduction

A young father-to-be found himself in the delivery room with his wife. The birth of his first child was obviously just minutes away. He kept saying to himself, "Why am I here? I'm completely useless for this kind of thing." More than once he fought back the urge to leave the room.

Through the blood and mess he could see the head of his son starting to come through. "Crowning," as he had been told in the childbirth preparation classes. Then, almost before he realized that it had happened, his child was out and a part of the world.

He'd been stifling a constant sense of panic throughout the labor and birth. He took one look at his new son, let out a scream that could be heard all over the maternity ward, and bolted from the room and out of the hospital.

He finally returned several hours later, quite ashamed of

1

himself, and quite drunk. He located the head nurse on the floor and made an attempt to explain his actions.

"I've been out drinking," he said, ". . . and thinking. I just couldn't face the fact that we had a deformed child. But I know that it's my responsibility, and now I'm prepared to do whatever is necessary."

The nurse was baffled by his speech at first. She took the father to the nursery and showed him a beautiful, nearly perfect baby boy.

The father was astounded. After all, he'd seen the baby come out. It had been a bluish-purple-gray, with an outrageously warped head and flattened face. It had looked like something out of a horror movie. Now here was this gorgeous baby boy with a name tag that showed that it was his own.

Although he'd gone to childbirth classes, no one had told him that a baby born vaginally is going to look a little strange for a while. The doctor knew. The nurse knew. His wife had at least some idea. The father didn't.

In some ways that story (yes, it *is* a true story) is rather amusing. In other ways it's sad, because it shows how far out of things Dad has been, and not by choice. A few decades ago that story couldn't have happened because the father wouldn't have been allowed in the delivery room. Now he is not just allowed to be in the delivery room, he is often encouraged to be there. That's a big step forward, but it's still just one step.

Like more than 85 percent of all fathers, the father in the story truly wanted to be involved with the birth of his child. He had no idea what to do, or how to do it. He felt lost. But he realized that the child is just as much his as it is the mother's. He wanted to be a part. His greatest problem was that he didn't have access to the information he needed. Even with the present trend of encouraging the father to take part, he had a hard time finding any complete and reliable sources of information that are meant for him. Out of hundreds of books on pregnancy, birth, and child care, a very few are written with Dad in mind. Many don't even mention the father.

The new father might find himself feeling left out and unimportant—almost unwanted. Because of this, many fathers don't ask questions. It's common for the father to feel that he is ignorant, and to feel a little foolish. Unfortunately, it's not unusual for him to be *made* to feel this way. This is especially true of the first-time father, but can also include the man who already has two, three, or more children.

Throughout his upbringing and education, chances are good that he has been given only the most basic information about conception, pregnancy, birthing, and care of the child. He might have even been told something like, "This is none of the father's business. Pregnancy is a purely female concern that males cannot hope to understand."

For many generations men had been kept out in the name of "morality," and from the assumption that they were, by nature, ignorant in such matters, incapable of understanding, and that they just didn't care. Just about anything and everything dealing with reproduction was kept in the hands of the women. The man didn't belong. Once he'd "planted his seed," he was no longer needed other than to provide financial support. The man might father a number of children without ever being a part of the process. Men were kept out. In one case, a German doctor was burned to death at the stake after he disguised himself as a woman so he could witness a birthing firsthand.

Medicine progressed. Things began to change. As the medical profession grew, it became male-dominated. Since being pregnant and giving birth can be considered a medical condition, around the turn of this century the medical profession began to squeeze out the midwives. By 1930 laws against widwifery were being passed in many states. The attitude was that anyone without proper medical training had no business being around someone in a "medical condition."

The midwives were pushed out, and were sometimes even thrown into jail.

Simultaneously only a relatively few women managed to become medical doctors. This wasn't because they were incapable but because of social attitudes. Consequently, decades passed in which women were being moved out of the labor and delivery rooms. That even began to include the mother herself. By the 1940s and 1950s a few doctors were saying that they wished they could figure out a way to keep even the mother out of the delivery room. She got in the way.

It was often assumed that she wouldn't be capable of understanding, so she was rarely informed about what was happening. It became common practice to give the mother potent drugs during labor and birth, to keep her out of the medical procedure of birthing. New drugs were discovered. They did a variety of things, from knocking the mother out (anesthetics) to keeping her fully conscious but making her forget the pain afterward (amnesiacs).

When "the time" came, Mom was rushed to the hospital. She was taken away from those she loved and trusted, and was placed in a ward or semiprivate room with other women going through the same thing, all of them on anesthetics or amnesiacs. Control of what was happening was taken from her. It was also taken away from the one she relied on and trusted most—her husband and the father.

Dad was shoved into a tiny room to wait with the other fathers. He sat nervously, staring at the foreboding sign NO FATHERS ALLOWED BEYOND THIS POINT.

It was "modern" to have a drug-controlled birth, and "modern" to use a scientific bottle-fed formula instead of breast-feeding. It was "modern" to do a variety of things that have since been shown to be potentially detrimental to the mother, to the child, and to the family unit. Many of you reading this were possibly brought into the world in just this way.

The drugs used *sometimes* caused permanent harm, but

even when they didn't, they often robbed the mother of one of the most incredible experiences a person can have. (That's not a male perspective, it's echoed by a very large number of mothers.) Also, despite efforts to make them complete, the scientific formulae poured into the bottles for baby just didn't quite have everything that baby needed. In short, the "modern" hospital procedures weren't what the mother, the child—or the father—needed.

Then a movement began to put the mother back into her proper place. Instead of forcing drugs on her, she was encouraged to relax and let the event occur more naturally—to allow her body to do the job. More, efforts were made to inform and educate the mother so that she could play that important role and understand.

During the past couple of decades, the mother and child have been moving back into their deserved and needed first place. Literally hundreds of books have been written for pregnant women and new mothers. Some magazines are completely dedicated to it; others have a heavy concentration on it.

Studies show what is only logical and to be expected. When the mother is well informed, and when the mystery of pregnancy and birth is removed, everything goes much more smoothly. There are far fewer complications. And this is just the doctor's perspective. For the mother herself, the more she knows and understands, the better she can handle, and enjoy, the experience. The more she knows, the better things are for everyone.

Exactly the same is true for the father. The more the father is kept ignorant and out of it, the more likely it is that there will be problems. Contrarily, the more he knows, the better he'll be able to be involved, and again everyone benefits—during the pregnancy, during the birth, and afterward.

AMA statistics show that a woman undergoing pregnancy and birth while the father is there by her side all along is far less likely to have complications. (There are also far fewer malpractice suits, which could be at least one of the reasons that fathers are being encouraged more and more to be a part of it.)

After the birth . . . well, a father who has been there to watch his child being born, and who holds that child in his arms moments after the birth, can't help but be moved. Instead of being "her child" it becomes "*our* child."

The family unit becomes stronger and more secure. It's not unusual for the couple to feel much closer together. Divorce rates go down. The child is raised in a more stable home, which is well known to produce a happier, more successful person.

What it comes down to is that there are only benefits in getting involved. With the mysteries gone, you begin to recognize that you're much more than just "planting the seed." The man and the woman have brought a new life into the world *together*. It takes a female *and* a male. For every mother there is a father.

The signs in hospitals (NO FATHERS BEYOND THIS POINT) are coming down. The attitudes are following, although more slowly. Dad isn't just being allowed to go into the delivery room, he's being encouraged to do so. To repeat, about 85 percent of all fathers now become closely involved with the pregnancy and birthing. More than 60 percent attend the births of their children. This is significant, especially when you consider only a very few employers have any kind of paternity leave.

The truth is, most fathers *want* to be involved. Some more than others, to be sure, but your desire to be a real part of the pregnancy, the birthing, and the lives of your children isn't unusual. Pregnancy comes about only when there is *both* a mother and a father. The importance of that simple fact goes far beyond mere biology.

It's not unusual for the new father to feel reluctant, and even a little afraid. You may find yourself having doubts about your ability to be a good father. And there is likely to be at least some resistance as you try to become involved. I faced all these myself, which is at least part of the reason I was married for fourteen years before my son was born.

After he was born, the fears remained, but I refused to give in. The actual effects didn't sink in until a few days later. My wife was resting in the bedroom while I cooked dinner and cleaned the kitchen. Out in the garage was a swinging crib I'd built, with the last coat of varnish drying. As I mopped the floor I heard my wife laughing and went back to find out why.

She said, "Don't you realize that you were singing?"

No, I hadn't noticed. Nor had I noticed how much fun I was having at being a new father. Even mopping the floor wasn't work—it was being involved. It was being a father.

Orders of Importance

The child obviously comes first. A very close second is the mother. Especially during the pregnancy and birthing, what affects one affects the other.

Mom's body grows the child, provides all the nutrition, protects it, and pushes it out into the world. Her role is primary, and should remain that way from before conception through (at least) the first months of the baby's life. Nothing is more important than Mom and the child at this time. Mother/child should be—*must* be—first priority.

Then comes Dad. What the father does, or does not do, affects the mother and child. Without his support and love, Mom's attitude going into birth will be worsened. Without his love and support afterward, neonatal care can be difficult, verging on impossible. His support at the birth itself can make all the difference between the need for anesthetic and/or surgery and a smooth and easy birth. After the birth, the importance of his love, support, and participation will continue for decades to come.

Think of a woman giving birth all alone. Compare this to a woman going through the same thing, but while being surrounded by those who love and care for her. The person most appropriate for that role is you, the father. You are more important than you might realize.

"Support" doesn't mean just paying the bills, it means being there. It means being a real part of things. During the pregnancy and birthing, your role can be critical. After the birth, you move from third place to a primary role shared with the mother.

Parenthood is a partnership. At least it can be, and should be. During the pregnancy and birthing, the well-being of the mother and child are paramount. When the child is born, the parents become more and more equal in the importance of their roles. Even if Mom is breast-feeding, there's nothing preventing the father from giving a bottle while Mom rests. You are certainly just as capable of changing a diaper, giving a bath, or rocking your child to sleep.

Yes, Dad, you *are* important.

What Can You Expect?

The pregnancy can be a trying time. The mother's body, and her hormones, change. She might say and do what seem to be strange things. If you know ahead of time what to expect, that time can be easier for both of you. This helps you to provide the understanding needed.

One young mother woke her husband in the middle of the night and said that she couldn't sleep. He flipped on the light and noticed some spots of blood on the sheet. This turned out to be normal spotting caused by the pelvic examination performed earlier in the day, but the father didn't know this, and she'd forgotten that the doctor had told her it might happen. The end result was a rush to the hospital.

The panic could have been avoided if the father (and the mother) had been better informed.

Mom will have complaints. Her legs swell up. Foods might taste funny, sometimes to the point of nausea. Later, her sleep could be interrupted by a kick from inside. Throughout you'll face her mood swings. (Recognize that she can't control most of these.)

There will be doctor's appointments. Lots of them! These will come closer and closer together as the "due date" is approached. Some of these will be intimate in nature. Mom and the doctor might not want you around. Most of the exams are more mundane. Attend if you can. (There's nothing quite like hearing the heartbeat of your unborn child.)

There are decisions to be made concerning the birth. Will Mom receive any drugs? Which ones? What are the benefits compared to harmful side effects? What complications can arise, and what will be done? Does the doctor automatically perform an episiotomy and why? (Or why not?) What about circumcision if the child is a boy?

The decisions on many of these things are of more direct concern to the mother than to the father, but this doesn't mean that the father should stay out of the decisions. If he's informed and takes an active part, his input can be very important. The final decision will still often be hers, but she won't be making it alone. And whatever decision she makes, he'll know what's going on.

There is no way to predict when or how the child will come. Only about 5 percent are born on the due date. It's not unusual for the event to happen days or weeks ahead of that date. If it goes much beyond, the doctor will probably induce labor. About the best you can do is to expect the unexpected.

There are a number of conditions that are common with a newborn. For example, jaundice is one of the most common neonatal (new birth) conditions. Mom may or may not know how minor it usually is. The uninformed Dad almost never knows, because he has never been told. He could hear,

"Your baby has jaundice and needs bilirubin treatments," and go into an instant panic. The informed father will know that this is quite common and involves little more than placing the child under a light to help stimulate skin pigments.

This happened when Danny was born. It was time for us to check out and go home. We were dressed, packed, and ready to leave, and waited only for our new son to be brought to us. After some waiting we pressed the call button. The nurse told us it would be just a few more minutes. After another forty-five minutes we pressed the button again. This time the nurse told us that there was a problem, but she couldn't tell us what it was without the doctor's permission, and he was temporarily unavailable.

After another hour of waiting and not knowing just what was wrong, I finally demanded to know. We were told curtly, "Your child has jaundice." There was no explanation about what this meant. Fortunately, we'd taken the time to learn (and had an excellent physician willing to answer any and all questions).

More and more, people are demanding personal participation in their medical care, including during pregnancy and the birth of their children. If a particular doctor or hospital still follows the ridiculous idea that the mother and father have no rights, the pregnant couple can, and should, go elsewhere to get the kind of treatment that they need and deserve. It's better for the mother. It's better for the father. And it's better for your new child.

Getting Involved

No matter how you look at it, there is every reason to get involved, and no reason at all to stay silently on the sidelines. It is quickly becoming more accurate to say, "*We* are having a baby," rather than "She is having a baby."

Many fathers *do* want to get involved. You're certainly

not alone. In fact, those fathers who don't try to get involved are in a 15 percent minority (which includes times when the father isn't even known).

You're also not alone if you feel left out, unwanted, out of place, and even a little stupid. This can make fathers feel afraid to get involved, despite their desire to do so. Even those fathers who attend childbirth classes experience a reluctance when it comes time to attend the actual birth.

Mom has an abundance of material available, all written with *her* in mind, to inform *her*. This is as it should be.

Dad has literally nothing. He has nowhere to go, and nothing to fall back on. My own research during my wife's pregnancy revealed that there were very few books for the father, with most being inadequate. Even in childbirth classes, the vast majority of the information is aimed at the mother. (Again, this is as it should be—but it does have the effect of leaving Dad feeling lost.) In conducting interviews for this book, it wasn't unusual for the father to say that the instructor would put humor into the class by poking fun at the fathers.

As the average dad goes through school, he is given the rough basics, if that much. It's not at all unusual for the male to enter into marriage and to start raising a family with very little real knowledge about reproduction, and even less about pregnancy, childbirth, and neonatal care.

Some say that the father's presence is enough, and that is true within limits. Even a relatively uneducated father can be of great help by simply letting his wife squeeze his hand during the birth. Some—unfortunately including some childbirth educators—seem quite happy with just this. One noted film, for example, spends an hour talking about parent-child bonding. In that hour is a twenty-two-second scene showing a father holding his baby, with the narrator saying, ". . . and the father can bond with his children, too." End of scene, and once more the father disappeared, not to be seen again until the closing credits rolled.

Childbirth classes concentrate on the mother, as they should, but often neglect to give the father any of the specific information about *his* role. One father who faithfully attended the classes reported that every time he asked, "What should I do?" he was answered with a vague, "Everything you can." If he pressed with, "Such as?" the response was, "Anything the mother needs."

Without the information and knowledge, how can he take an effective part? How can he help to make intelligent decisions, or even to take an intelligent part? He can stand there feeling lost and helpless and be the bumbling father right out of the comic strips. Or he can become more active and play his full role in the partnership called parenting.

Forearmed with some knowledge, you as the concerned father won't feel as helpless. You will find yourself the major source of strength for Mom. You can appreciate just what is happening. You can more thoroughly enjoy your new son or daughter.

You can also help to protect your wife and child, and to help in making critical decisions. Consider just the birth itself. There are many controversial methods and techniques used. The three most common examples are: an *episiotomy* (a surgical cut in the perineum), the use of an *analgesic* (such as Demerol, which is synthetic morphine) to ease pain, and the birthing position of the mother.

In the first case, many claim that the episiotomy is the best way to prevent painful and difficult-to-heal tearing of the tissues. Others say that this is the single most abused and unneeded surgical procedure in America. Which do you believe, and why? It could be that an episiotomy *is* necessary in your particular case, but will you know if it is? Or is it being done merely as a routine for the convenience of the doctor (and the inconvenience of the mother)?

Demerol and other drugs are used to "take off the edge" of the pain in the majority of births. But did you know, or has the doctor told you, that Demerol is used in other types of surgery to lessen or stop muscle spasms? Or that Mom needs those spasms to get the baby out? You (and Mom) are told that the drug won't affect the baby, and will do nothing but make the birth easier. Others point to evidence that *any* drug will get into the baby and can cause complications. They also claim that the drug causes a more difficult and more lengthy labor in most cases and in more than a few cases has forced an emergency procedure, such as cesarean, because the mother's muscles relax too much and can't push out the baby. (One study indicates that "safe" drugs have caused a fourfold increase of cesarean births while also causing a dramatic increase in maternal and fetal trauma.) Are painkilling drugs routine? What are the dangers and risks? Are the risks low enough to be offset by the lessening of pain?

The most common birth position for the mother is flat on her back with her legs spread and strapped into stirrups. This has an advantage for the doctor, since he or she can see better and has more working room. In many cases, it's easier on both the mother and child because of this. Other times it makes the birthing more difficult and can cause complications. (It brings with it a disadvantage for the mother. Lying on her back that way forces her to push against gravity.)

Being informed of these and other matters will help you, and your partner, to make intelligent and informed decisions. Even if the choice is taken out of your hands, at least you'll know what to expect.

The average person thinks nothing of spending years in school to learn how to do a particular job, including four or more years of intensive education and training in college or trade school. It's not unusual for someone to spend weeks or months deciding which car or stereo to buy. Along comes the single most important role in his life, that of being a father, and many are left to learning how to do the job by trial and error, or having to "cram" late in the pregnancy, and then with few or no reliable sources of information.

Think about signing over to a stranger the safety and

well-being of your own body. "Do what you want, even if it's experimental." There are pieces of paper hanging on the doctor's wall with that person's name on them, but what kind of student was he or she really? Does this person *really* care about your feelings and Mom's, and the safety of mother and baby? (In fairness, they usually do.) Or is it another case of too busy attendants just getting the job done with a minimum of time and a maximum of profit?

You could be signing over the very lives of your wife and your children.

Can you REALLY take that step blindly?

Most people in this country still have their children in a hospital environment, so the book will concentrate on that scenario. Which route you choose will be your own (hopefully informed) decision. Just because this book uses the term "the doctor" doesn't necessarily mean that a CNM (a certified midwife with a nursing degree) isn't equally competent.

There are many, many choices and options. It has been justly said that no two births, and no two pregnancies, are alike. One pregnancy might go along smoothly, with Mom having no difficulties other than trying to find new ways to entice Dad to be a part of it. The next might have her raving at times like a maniac and throwing things for no apparent reason. Even anatomically, no two women (and no two men) are exactly alike.

What you will find in this book, and in any book, are generalities, plus some of the most common similarities and differences. It simply isn't possible to present *all* the possibilities in one book.

You are reading a book from a distant writer. There will be doctors, nurses, perhaps a midwife and other medical professionals. Advice could come pouring in from family and friends, including from those who consider themselves "experts" although they have never had a child. You know your partner better than anyone else. During the pregnancy it may not seem that way, but it is true. The basic guidelines you need are here. Beyond, fill in the gaps by what you already know about your partner and from the particular circumstances.

Pregnancy, birth, and raising the child can be one of the best times of your life, or one of the worst. More likely it will be a combination of the two. Mom can't help some of the things she does. *You* can.

That's your job.

The job of this book is to help you.

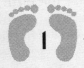

Some Basic Anatomy

$\mathcal{M}$ost of us had basic anatomy in school. Most fathers (and potential fathers) know at least some of the parts of the body—your own body and that of the mother. These basics, if you remember them, will take you a long way in the understanding of what is happening, why, and how. This knowledge can also help you to recognize and understand problems if they occur.

Don't let the technical nature of the terminology or of this chapter scare you. In most cases they'll make sense if you give them a chance. Your goal isn't to be working toward a degree in obstetrics, and there's no real need to be able to toss out all those fancy terms at will.

At the same time, the doctors, nurses, midwifes, etc.—and this book—will all be using that terminology. It's like anything else. When a field of knowledge uses specific terminology, it's to your benefit to become at least exposed to that terminology if you intend to understand. Although *dystocia* (difficult birth) or *puerperium* (the six weeks after the birth) aren't the kinds of words you're likely to encounter in usual daily life, you just might hear them while being a part of the pregnancy, birth, and recovery.

Don't worry too much about memorizing all the names and details. It won't hurt to do so, but it's not necessary. If you get into Chapter Six, for example, and just can't remember what the *areola* is, or if the doctor mentions a term you don't know, turn to the Glossary and look it up.

The purpose of this first chapter isn't to train you to be an obstetrician. It is merely to acquaint (or reacquaint) you with the basics of anatomy, and with the terminology used.

The Female Reproductive System

As a whole the female's external genitalia is called the *vulva* or *pudendum*. The *mons veneris* at the top consists of fatty tissue. This and the pubic bone beneath gives it a rounded appearance. Normally the opening to the vagina is partially closed off by the *labia* (Latin for "lips"). The larger, fleshier outer labia are the *labia majora* (easiest to remember as "major lips"). The outside is covered with hair, while the inside is smooth. Inside these labia is another pair of smaller folds of skin, the *labia minora* ("minor lips"), sometimes called the *nymphae*. During the birth the labia distend and are stretched to allow passage of the baby.

Beneath the top of the labia majora, and covered by a small hood (the *prepuce*) is the *clitoris*. This is analogous to the male's penis. The clitoris attains a degree of erection during sexual excitement, and has even been known to have its own type of ejaculation. Essentially it is the center of the female's sexual pleasure. With many women it is just barely visible even during a state of excitement.

About an inch beneath this and more or less inside the

labia minora is the *urethra*, from which the female urinates. This is also all but invisible in most women. Below the urethra is the opening to the vagina, or *introitus*. In most virgins and in many women who have not had a baby, the vaginal opening is kept partially closed by the *hymen*. Formerly there was the mistaken notion that an intact hymen signified that the woman was a virgin, and that one that was broken or absent meant she'd been sexually active. Today we know that any number of things can cause the hymen to break, and that in a few cases a hymen broken by intercourse can grow back. Regardless, what remains of this membrane, if anything, will rupture during the woman's first birth.

Between the bottom of the external genitalia and the anus is an area called the *perineum*. This area can become quite important during birth. Various hormones in Mom's body during labor cause the perineum to become softer and more flexible. Even so, having the baby's head pushing its way through an opening that is normally tight to the penis can cause a problem. It is quite common for the tissues of the perineum to tear. To reduce the risks of tearing, many physicians routinely make a surgical cut in the perineum, effectively creating a larger birth opening. This operation is called an episiotomy. The muscles are stitched together after the birth. It's not uncommon for the doctor to "overstitch," making the vaginal opening tighter and thus more pleasurable for the male during intercourse.

The vagina is a muscular and (fortunately) elastic tube that leads inward from the external genitalia to the uterus. During intercourse it stretches to accept a penis of just about any size, while still putting pressure and friction on the penis, thus stimulating ejaculation. During birth it stretches and expands to allow passage of the baby. Afterward it goes back into shape (or can be made to go back into shape through exercise).

A few inches inside the vagina is a conical structure about one inch long called the *cervix*. The cervix is the neck of the uterus. The outer portion of the cervix can be felt, and examined, with a finger inserted into the vagina. During pelvic exams the doctors and nurses will be checking the condition of the cervix, which gives them a clue as to when the baby will be coming and if there are complications.

During prepregnant intercourse, the sperm make their way through a hole in the cervix called the *os*. Once the woman is impregnated, a plug of mucous forms and the cervix closes off the uterus, allowing a sterile environment in which the fetus can develop. Not long before the birth, the mucous plug breaks loose. The cervix then begins to soften and thin out *(efface)*, and will eventually begin to open *(dilate)*. As mentioned above, in the final weeks, and just prior to the birth, the doctors and nurses will be regularly examining the cervix by touch to check how soft it has become and how dilated.

One of the things that seems to amaze most new parents is just how wide the dilatation becomes. In the final stages, the cervix will all but disappear, leaving a hole with a diameter of about four inches. This allows the baby to pass down through the cervix and into the birth canal (the vagina) and eventually out into the world and into your arms.

On the far side of the cervix is the uterine cavity—the *uterus*. This is a muscular organ, with a shape somewhat like an inverted pear, and a nonpregnant size of roughly two inches by two inches, with a one-inch cervical neck between the uterine body and the vagina. The walls are about the same thickness as your finger at the thinner parts and just shy of two fingers' thickness at the wider parts. The uterus is held in place by four pairs of ligaments, and also by the pelvic floor (the perineum).

As the fetus develops and grows, the uterus expands to allow the growth. The *placenta* develops where the fertilized egg implants itself, and the various fetal membranes grow. By the end of the pregnancy, the placenta will weigh more than a pound. It has to be "delivered" (removed) after the baby has been born, which is why it is then called the *after-birth*. Between the placenta and the fetus is a cord, the *umbilical cord*, which provides transport for everything the fetus needs.

Two "arms" stick out from the sides of the uterine cavity. These are the *fallopian tubes* or *oviducts*. Each is about four inches long. Their job is to "catch" the egg from the ovaries and carry it to the uterus.

The ovaries themselves are not physically attached to the fallopian tubes, but are usually close enough for the eggs to make the transfer successfully. Each of the two ovaries is about the size of the first joint of your little finger.

The eggs (*ova* as plural, and *ovum* as singular) develop inside the ovaries and are released one at a time (normally) on a monthly basis. This is the *menses*, coming from "month," more commonly called menstruation. You will probably also know it as a period (because it's periodic).

Conception

By the time the girl reaches puberty, her ovaries contain approximately four hundred thousand ova, each surrounded by a layer of *epithelioid granulosa* cells. The egg plus this layer is the *primordial follicle*. Only about 0.1 percent of these develop enough to create an egg capable of becoming another human being. (Of the four hundred thousand follicles, only about 450 manage to expel from the ovum.) Usually the female produces one egg per month for a period of roughly thirty-five years, at which time she reaches menopause. The remaining primordial follicles degenerate, and the female can no longer produce offspring.

About fourteen days before the beginning of the menstrual period, and twelve to sixteen days after the last period, another egg will have developed sufficiently—ripened—to erupt (almost literally) from the ovary, where it is picked up by the fallopian tube and funneled toward the uterus. Not too far from the ovary is a section of the fallopian tube called the *ampule*. In almost all cases, this is where the egg is waiting and is where fertilization takes place.

The so-called rhythm method of contraception (or conception, depending on what you're trying to do) is based on this cycle. The amount of time when fertilization is possible is actually quite short. If the sperm doesn't meet up with the egg within about forty-eight hours after the egg leaves the ovary, it will be too late. The ovum generally doesn't remain viable beyond about twenty-four hours, and although some sperm are still viable for as long as seventy-two hours, most die in the first twenty-four hours. Somewhere in the middle of the menstrual cycle is a period of two days or less during which the female tends to be fertile. (This period can't be accurately predicted, however, as those who use the rhythm method often find out when they are trying to have a baby, or when an unexpected pregnancy comes along.)

A literal flood of sperm starts working its way inward in search of the egg. A large number of sperm are killed almost immediately by the naturally acidic conditions inside the female. As the sperm swim along, even more die. Many simply get lost, and more than a few are so immature or malformed in the first place that they don't get anywhere. For example, some will have two tails, and will be trying to swim in two directions at once. A precious few (relatively—there are still many thousands at this point) make it to the uterine cavity.

Now the flood divides. Some of the sperm travel up the left fallopian tube, while the others go up the right. An egg ready for fertilization is in only one of the two. Those sperm that go up the wrong tube don't find anything to fertilize. Of those that are in the correct tube, the vast majority will die along the way. Out of some four hundred million sperm cells of the ejaculation, two thousand or fewer actually make it to the egg.

Of the sperm that eventually do find the egg, all try their

best to get inside to fertilize it. Only one will achieve that goal. The coating of the ovum makes the job difficult enough. To make it possible, the head of the sperm secretes an enzyme (hyaluronidase) to allow the sperm to burrow its way in. Once a single sperm manages to do this, the ovum "closes up," making it impossible for other sperm to penetrate.

The tail of the successful sperm falls off, leaving only the head. This head almost immediately begins to swell. After a while the twenty-three chromosomes of the male pronucleus will unite with the twenty-three chromosomes of the female pronucleus—and you have pregnancy.

The total journey made by the sperm is roughly five inches, and takes approximately thirty to forty minutes.

The fertilized and growing egg is moved down the tube by *cilia* (little "hairs") and a weak current in the fluid caused by the cilia. Within about three days the fertilized egg moves into the uterus, where it implants itself (within about four more days) and begins to develop into your new child.

The Breasts

The female breast has long been treated as a sexual object, perhaps because it has to do with child rearing (breast-feeding), just as the genitals have to do with childbirth. There are any number of theories as to why men are attracted to women's breasts (and why women are often every bit as sensitive about size, shape, etc.). A woman going topless in public is likely to be arrested. Breast-feeding in public is still frowned upon in most circles. The woman is usually expected to find a place to hide, even if her breasts are completely covered, so as not to offend.

Gray's Anatomy refers to breasts as "accessory glands of the generative system," which is exactly what they are. If you and your mate decide to breast-feed your child, you'll soon come to marvel at the capabilities of the breasts. They are capable of providing everything the baby needs to grow strong and healthy, and in just the right quantity. They even produce a substance high in protein and calories at the start, just when baby needs it most.

During pregnancy you'll almost certainly notice a change in Mom's breasts. Due to secretions of hormones such as estrogen, they'll become larger, and very likely will also become sensitive, possibly painful, and may even become itchy. This will go away, generally by the fourth month. It may also come back again after the birth, and will once again go away. However, it does mean that there will be a period of time in which you may have to be careful when touching them, or even when giving Mom a needed and deserved hug.

As the breasts increase in size, they also get heavier. The tendency to sag becomes greater. This will continue through the pregnancy and beyond the weaning of the baby. Most women find that they are more comfortable wearing a supportive bra during this time, even if they're not used to wearing a bra at all normally. The practice is beneficial in any case since it will help to decrease the sagging later on and can also prevent stains on clothing from the small leaks that the breasts will have.

The appearance of silvery-white streaks called *striae,* or stretch marks, is common. The second name is unfortunate and misleading. It comes from the fact that when someone gains weight and size in some part of the body, the skin is stretched, sometimes causing striae. And this is partially the cause of the striae on the breasts and elsewhere on Mom's body. But they are also caused by the increase in hormones in her body, which in turn causes a breakdown of protein.

Some have suggested the use of Vitamin E, both internally and as a massage oil, but there is no solid evidence that this will lessen the marks. In time the marks fade somewhat. They'll probably never disappear entirely.

In many women the *areola*—the colored area around the nipple—dramatically enlarges and becomes darker during pregnancy. In some cases it will become almost black. This fades in time, particularly after breast-feeding has been stopped. The increase in size and darkening in color is one sign of pregnancy, especially a first pregnancy.

There have been cases in which the woman will rush to the doctor because a number of small bumps have appeared around the areola. In actuality, this is a perfectly normal occurrence. The bumps are *Montgomery's tubercles,* which have always been there but which tend to be more obvious when the woman is pregnant. In some cases the increase in size causes the woman to fear breast cancer.

Later on, after the child is born, and especially if Mom is breast-feeding, the breasts will grow even larger and fill with milk. Overfilling can cause problems at first, but an amazing thing happens for the breast-feeding mother. After a very short time, the breasts will settle down to a routine. They'll produce just the right amount of milk for the baby's needs, with a quality of nutrition that can't be beat by anything that even the most advanced scientific laboratories can produce.

What is surprising to many men (and many women) is that breast size has little to do with the ability to breast-feed. Whether your mate is a 40D or a 32A, she can probably still provide for the child. Breast size is not an accurate gauge of whether Mom can breast-feed. The woman can fit the classic description of being "flat as a board" and still be wonderfully adept at, and capable of, breast-feeding. Another might be "voluptuous" and find that she has to use bottle-feeding as a supplement or entirely.

Growth of the breasts from puberty is caused by various estrogens. During pregnancy the placenta releases additional estrogen, which in turn causes more development of the milk-carrying ducts, hence the tenderness and increase in size. Progesterone causes further development of the alveoli. Toward the end of pregnancy, prolactin, from the anterior pituitary gland, works with the other hormones to stimulate the final development to prepare the breasts to feed the new baby.

The inside of the breast contains a large number of milk-producing nodules. Each network of milk-producing nodules leads to its own outlet in the nipple. It takes some skill and experience to be able to express that milk by hand, but the baby's mouth is absolutely perfect for the job. It certainly won't take the baby long to learn how to do it. Babies even have a built-in reflex—called the *rooting reflex*—that causes them to automatically turn to the breast and start sucking in just the right way.

What helps in this respect is the release of the hormone *oxytocin* from the pituitary. As baby suckles, nerve impulses trigger the production of oxytocin, which in turn causes muscular contractions. Once again, nature has provided the perfect solution to postpregnancy recuperation. The oxytocin will help the uterus and tummy in general to get back into shape. It also stimulates cells (the *myoepithelial cells*) around the milk-storing alveoli to contract, thus squeezing the milk out of the alveoli and into the ducts that carry the milk from the breast to the baby.

This process is called "letdown." That doesn't mean that Mom feels let down or depressed. It means that the milk is let down from the alveoli into the ducts.

If this doesn't happen, the alveoli store up the milk to the point that the breasts become overly full. This can be a problem when feedings are missed, if mothers are working, or when the baby takes to sleeping for longer periods of time. The breasts will become more tender, even painful, and the letdown reflex may be sluggish. (It will take a while before the milk begins to flow.) In more severe cases, it may not flow at all. It's possible that infection will set in *(mastitis)*. In both such cases, she may have to see the doctor. Generally, however, the mother produces the right amount of milk at the right time.

The first fluid produced is called *colostrum,* and is often called "early milk" since it begins to show up before the baby is born. It's also almost the entire breast output for the first few days of nursing.

Colostrum is said to contain the largest quantities of antibodies. You'll hear it said that if Mom does decide to bottle-feed, she should at least try to breast-feed the child for the first few days to help protect the baby. Within the first three days, the colostrum disappears and is replaced by the milk itself. The antibodies continue, of course, boosting the baby's immunity to disease, but the fat content in the milk goes up, along with increased levels of lactose, casein, and other nutrients and substances. (Colostrum has almost no fat content.)

Colostrum is just about perfect to meet the needs of the first days of a baby's life. Sit down and design THE perfect formula for a baby right after its birth, and you'll come up with something very much like colostrum.

Then, after a day or so, the baby's needs change. Mom's breasts make the changes automatically, and at just the right times. Not only that, the breast secretions are automatically sterile, come in precisely the right quantities, and increase in quantity as the baby grows so perfectly on that diet.

Hormones

In both the male and female, more comes into play than just the reproductive systems. The human body works as a whole, intricate unit. Change one part of that, and other changes take place elsewhere in the body. This overall situation is important in Mom, and increases in importance as she approaches the day of delivery.

Explaining how the hormones work and what they do

isn't easy. More often than not, a series of hormones are interlinked, with one stimulating production of another, which in turn stimulates something else. A single hormone can have a wide variety of functions, which are further increased as it reacts with, or against, other hormones. The subject is so complex that even the best experts often find themselves guessing.

What matters to you isn't a full understanding of the entire hormonal process, but what all this means to you, to your wife, and to your baby.

You'll almost certainly have some rough times during the pregnancy. Your otherwise perfectly sane mate might suddenly take to throwing things when you show up five minutes late (or five minutes early). She might cry when you bring home a box of chocolates—one day because you're sweet and considerate, and the next because you're making her fat. Then she might scream at you the next day for not bringing them home because now you're ignoring her.

You might find that her sex drive has taken a sudden swing upward so that she seems insatiable. (This is thought to be caused, at least in part, by increased estrogen.) Or you might find yourself leading the life of a monk for a while. Either way, depending on how the hormones swing, her mood can shift from day to day, or even faster.

Those are extremes. But not too extreme. They happen. Uncontrollable reactions on the part of the mother are common. They are, however, usually more moderate. The idea that a pregnant woman becomes like an insane person is largely false and entirely unfair.

It's important to keep in mind that she often can't help herself. Her body is going through a variety of changes. You can see the physical changes. You can't see the hormonal changes that are going on inside. You can massage her legs and back to relieve the pains and swelling, but there isn't a thing you can do about the hormones. Even the best doctors and scientists don't completely understand what happens, why it happens, or what exactly all the hormones do.

The *gonadotropic* hormones come from the anterior pituitary gland. These are follicle-stimulating hormone (called FSH) and lutenizing hormone (LH). These hormones are responsible for the reproductive cycle. In the female's very young years, the hormones are almost totally absent. Then, when she reaches about eight years of age, the pituitary starts kicking out more and more of these hormones. By the time she reaches an age between eleven to fifteen, they have caused the onset of the sexual cycle. Puberty. And she can become pregnant. This process continues throughout her reproductive life, and governs the menstrual cycle and ovulation.

There seems to be evidence that HCG (*human chorionic gonadotropin*) stimulates the production of progesterone. There is also a possible link between HCG and morning sickness. The quantity of HCG increases after the fifth week of pregnancy, hitting a peak somewhere around the eighth week. This also happens to be when morning sickness is at its worst.

There are two basic categories of hormone that are secreted by the ovaries. These are the estrogens and the progesterones. Both are responsible for a wide variety of effects. Not all of these are understood.

Estrogen is sometimes called the female sex hormone since it is responsible for secondary sexual characteristics and for the monthly menstrual cycle. This, and a variety of other effects brought about by the estrogen group, make it an important hormone.

The amount of estrogen increases in the pregnant female. (Birth control pills are essentially estrogenic and make the body think it's pregnant by increasing the amount of estrogen in the body.) This causes a number of things to happen—some good and some not so good.

For example, the increased estrogen stimulates the

breasts and begins the preparation for breast-feeding. Consequently, the breasts enlarge. (They often become overly sensitive, at least for a while, so don't be surprised if your wife doesn't want you to touch her, or even to hug.)

The increased level also causes sodium to bind water, which in turn causes water retention, edema (swelling), even headaches. There also seem to be links between estrogen and breast cancer, which originally caused some experts to warn that birth control pills increase the incidence of breast cancer. (Recent evidence indicates the reverse, that birth control pills or pregnancy reduces the incidence of breast cancer. The findings are not complete at this point.)

Normally estrogen peaks at the time of ovulation. Progesterone sits level through most of the menstrual cycle, begins a sharp climb at the onset of ovulation, hits a peak at about day twenty-two of the cycle, and by day twenty-eight and the end of the cycle, has dropped back to a low and steady level again.

Progesterone is also a so-called female hormone, and is sometimes called the pregnancy hormone, and even the "baby hormone."

It is naturally manufactured in the *corpus luteum* (a body that develops in the egg-producing follicle in the ovary after the follicle ruptures and releases the egg) of the ovaries, in the adrenal glands, and by the placenta. An inadequate level of progesterone has been linked with miscarriage. This created the idea of giving the mother doses of progesterone during pregnancy to reduce the risk of miscarriage.

It didn't take long before the profession realized that this procedure brought with it the tendency to cause sometimes severe birth defects, especially when synthetic progesterone was used. Even natural progesterone is now administered very carefully and only in dire need. Many doctors won't use it at all, or will restrict the use to encouraging conception. (This is generally done either with suppositories or, more commonly, with intramuscular injections of something called 17-hydroxy-progesterone, a chemical that helps to stimulate natural progesterone production and activity, which in turn helps to get the conception to "take.")

Important Skeletal Structures

Obviously, all the bones of the body are important. Those of the *pelvis* play the primary role in childbirth.

The pelvis is shaped like a ringed basin with a hole in the middle that is partially blocked by a tapering structure as the spine comes to an end. The pelvic area is made up of a central structure, a pair of large bones toward the top, a smaller pair toward the bottom, and a bony arch toward the front, with these last two forming small circles.

The spine joins to and is supported by the lesser, or true, pelvis. This part curves and tapers down to the *sacrum* and *coccyx* (the "tailbone"). It is joined at both sides to the hipbones.

The hipbones are technically called the *ilium* and are the major parts of the greater, or false, pelvis. The top curve is the *iliac crest*. Toward the bottom they become the *ischium* and the *pubis*. These are actually separate bones that are flexible in a newborn. Later the joints solidify.

On the inside of the ischium are small bumps, called *ischial spines*. These can play an important part in childbirth. Large ischial spines can effectively decrease the size of the pelvic outlet (see below), which is the hole through which the baby must travel to get out. They can also cause physical injury (temporary) to the baby.

The pubic arch peaks at another joint, the *pubic symphysis*. This is the hard bone just above the vaginal area. The distance between the pelvic arch and the sacrum and coccyx makes up the *pelvic outlet*. The doctor will measure this to be sure that the baby has sufficient room to get out. (See Chapter Two.) In a few cases the outlet is too small, which means that at best Mom may have a difficult birth. If small enough, a C-section may be necessary. Fetal size can become even more important in such cases and will be monitored.

It may not seem like it at first, but the skeletal structure of the baby's skull is also highly important, particularly the top (vertex) of the skull.

The baby's skull consists of a number of bones held together at flexible joints by membranes. The joints later ossify and harden to make the skull, in effect, a single, hard structure. If the skull were completely hard at birth, very few babies would make it out without medical intervention.

The flexible nature of the bones of the baby's skull allow the skull to mold and shape as it passes through the birth canal. Although the mother's pelvic bones and joints are somewhat flexible in themselves, this is rarely enough. The baby's skull must also flex and mold. Shortly after the birth, the bones move back into their normal positions. The odd shape of the head immediately after the birth, caused by the molding, will soon disappear.

The top front of the head *(sinciput)* has two frontal bones. Immediately behind these is the *anterior fontanelle*. This is one of the two major soft spots on a baby's head. It's large enough that complete hardening takes some time.

Behind that are the two *parietal bones,* later attached to the frontal bones at the *coronal suture*. The parietal bones are large structures that cover much of the head. They join at the top in the middle at the *sagittal suture*. During birth, the two frontal bones may actually slide beneath these two larger bones.

Still moving toward the back is the *posterior fontanelle,* another soft spot that tends to remain for a while. The back of the skull *(occiput)* is made up of the occipital bone, which joins to the parietal bones at the lambdoidal suture.

As already mentioned, the flexibility of the baby's skull— and the mother's pelvic bones—is important during the birth. Once again, if your wife gives birth vaginally, expect to see at least some molding. The baby's head will seem deformed. The head will take its normal shape soon afterward.

The process of ossification of the skull takes a while. Longer for the fontanelles since they are larger. This means that you must be careful handling the newborn. The head is a sensitive area in any case. Until the joints of the skull bones become hard, it's even more sensitive. That doesn't mean that you should be afraid to stroke your baby's head, just that you should exercise a little extra caution.

What Can You Do?

In general, there's nothing to do. Anatomy is anatomy. There's nothing you can do to make her pelvis larger or more flexible. You can mention behavior shifts you think might be due to hormones, but there's nothing you can do but put up with the quirks.

Small shifts, small changes, can be and usually should be largely ignored. Your primary concern is to know enough so that more drastic changes are noticed. Some swelling, especially around the ankles, can be expected. If it becomes severe, and especially if it becomes painful for her, bring it up.

Mostly, the best you can do is to learn as much as you can about the physical and psychological aspects—but keep in mind that you are *not* a doctor. Don't fall into the trap of thinking you know more than you really do.

At the same time, the more you know, the better you will be able to spot potential problems, and possible medical errors.

2

The Beginnings

*T*he first few months of pregnancy—the first trimester—are undramatic in most cases. There are signs of pregnancy, but most of them are subtle and can often go unnoticed. It's not unusual for the pregnancy to be two or even three months along before it's noticed. Sooner or later more definite signs will appear, until eventually it's obvious to anyone that something is going on.

Some people sit back and wait for the really obvious physical signs. By then the pregnancy might have progressed halfway through full term. In this case, there's not much time left to take care of all the details. Worse, growth and development of the fetus may have been affected by bad habits, and health problems for Mom can have set in. As a general rule, the earlier you know for sure about the pregnancy, the better.

Even a healthy woman needs more care during a pregnancy. The doctor is likely to prescribe prenatal vitamins and perhaps changes in her diet. If she is on medication of some kind, it may be changed. Remember that during this time literally everything she eats, drinks, or does can affect both the mother and the new life inside her body. Beyond this, there are many things coming that require planning, or that at the very least will go easier when you have more time. (See also Chapters Three and Four on preparing for the birth.)

It is nearly useless to see a doctor for diagnosis too early. Every possible sign or symptom could have an alternate explanation. The chances for a misdiagnosis increase. The exam and tests might indicate pregnancy when none exists; or the tests could be negative even though Mom is pregnant. (This certainly includes the "at home" tests. These are fine as a rough indicator, by the way, but should be followed up by a professional examination.)

Is She Pregnant?

This question, or its answer, can come as a shock, or as wonderful news, depending on your point of view. Of course, if you've purposely planned for the child and have just as purposely made the attempt, your sense of anxiety will be quite different from that of the couple who aren't quite so sure that they want a baby.

Either way, it's a question virtually every man (and woman, obviously) faces sooner or later. Since this book is concerned with parenting, I'll make the assumption that Mom coming back with, "I'm pregnant!" will be one of the great thrills of your life. (If it isn't, hang in there until you see your child born, until you've held that child a few times, or perhaps until you hear "Daddy" for the first time.)

Chances are good that Mom will already know if she is pregnant. There are "internal" indicators. Mom can usually feel them. Some of these seem to border on psychic. More than a few will-be-mothers "feel" that they are pregnant. The doctor merely verifies the fact and begins the long process of making sure that everything runs smoothly. Be aware, however, that more than a few women are so determined to become pregnant that they truly think they are, and even show all the signs, when they are not pregnant at all.

A first outward indication is that Mom no longer has periods (a condition called *amenorrhea*). A period is basically the sloughing off of an ovum (egg) that hasn't been fertilized, won't become a child, and is of no further use.

Menstruation, or lack of it, is actually a fairly poor early indicator. It becomes an even worse indicator if her periods have been inconsistent in the past, either in regularity or in intensity. Amenorrhea can also be brought on by stress, illness, a change in environment or conditions, poor diet, sudden weight loss, stopping oral contraception, and a variety of other reasons.

On the other end of things, it's quite common for a pregnant woman to continue to have periods for a short time even though she is pregnant. Almost always these are shorter in duration, with less-than-usual bleeding, but they may be strong enough and long enough so that you won't know for certain.

At about three to four weeks after conception, many women feel a tingling sensation in their breasts. By six weeks the breasts may begin to enlarge and become sensitive to the touch. The breasts might also change in appearance, with surface veins possibly beginning to show. As discussed in Chapter One, little nodules (Montgomery's tubercles, or glands) might appear around the nipples, giving them a mottled, bumpy look.

A little later (at about sixteen weeks) the areola, the colored ring around the nipple, may expand and become darker. It's also possible that a secondary areola will develop. A little later (after a few months), the breasts may begin to leak a clear liquid (colostrum, or "early milk"), or this substance can be expressed manually.

About 50 percent of all pregnant women will have morning sickness, usually starting somewhere between four and fourteen weeks. These symptoms can often be mistaken for the flu, or even hunger. Nobody is quite sure what causes this, and there is no valid cure. Sometimes a light meal first thing in the morning will help. Saltine crackers are a classic "cure." If the condition persists or is excessive, don't take any chances. See the doctor as soon as possible. Severe morning sickness can be a bad sign.

Other indicators are changes in appetite (including cravings), tiredness, increased urination, the appearance of a darkish line from the pubic area to the navel (linea nigra), and even an early and slight bulge. As with the other signs and symptoms, all of these can have other explanations.

Assuming that she is pregnant, the due date is predicted by adding seven days to the first day of the last period, then subtracting three months. This works out to 280 days (forty weeks), which is considered the average. It's called gestational age, which is actually about two weeks off from the conceptual age. In other words, if the gestational age is eight weeks, the actual age since conception is about six weeks.

It doesn't matter, though. The prediction serves only as a guideline. It's quite rare for a woman to actually have her child on the calculated due date. This happens only about 5 percent of the time. The other 95 percent of the time, she'll be early or late, often by several weeks. In fact, giving birth two weeks on either side of the due date is quite common, and it's not unusual for the calculation to be off by almost a month. In this case, however, there is possible reason for concern. Regular examinations during the pregnancy will usually show that the original calculations were off for a variety of reasons and the doctor will reassess the situation.

Chapters Three and Four discuss preparation. Read them carefully! And keep in mind that you might easily find yourself with a new baby a month or more earlier than expected. Or a month late. (Most doctors won't let it go more than two weeks over unless there is reason to believe that the original calculations were in error.)

First Visit to the Doctor

The ob-gyn exam room has been off-limits to most men (other than doctors) for years. While this protects the privacy and sensitivity of the female patient, it throws the other half of our population into the dark. Yet there's nothing dark or secretive about it.

When Mom goes to the doctor, one of the first things the doctor will ask is, "Why are you here?" What happens next depends at least in part on when she last visited that particular doctor. Many doctors will have a short conference with the mother to get to know her better and to get a more complete medical history. This discussion period also serves to help the female patient to relax. After all, she is about to go through a very intimate and somewhat uncomfortable examination.

The possibility of pregnancy, particularly when the patient is new, generally requires a very complete physical exam. This is to establish her general condition and to spot any early signs of potential trouble.

The doctor or the nurse will take and record the vitals—height, weight, blood pressure, heart rate, urinalysis, etc. Each of these is important immediately, and will also give a basis of comparison as things progress. A medical history will also be taken, to alert the doctor to possible complications and health conditions.

Mom will be directed to undress and to put on one of several varieties of gowns, towels, or covers.

Particularly if the patient hasn't seen the doctor for a while or is a new patient, the breasts will be examined. A visual exam comes first (and is usually so subtle and quick due to the doctor's experience that many women don't realize that it has been done) to look for obvious problems. Palpation (probing by touch) determines if any hidden problems exist. This also shows if the glandular tissue in preparation for breast-feeding has begun to grow. Depending on how far the pregnancy has come along, the doctor may also try to express (squeeze out, called "stripping") colostrum as an indicator of pregnancy and the beginnings of lactation (producing milk).

Palpation of the abdomen is one of the major tests and will continue throughout pregnancy. The condition of many internal organs can be determined in this way. Liver and gall bladder (both in the upper right), the spleen (upper left), and the two kidneys are examined. The midabdomen is then palpated in order to check the condition and position of the uterus. By the tenth week of pregnancy, the doctor's trained fingers can usually find the slight swelling, and will know the difference between a baby and a tumor. (The baby is softer and rounder.)

The doctor may also listen for the fetal heartbeat and for other sounds—another item that goes into the regular checkups throughout pregnancy. It's unlikely that you will attend this first exam because it is often perceived as personal, and embarrassing. But go to the others if possible, and be sure to listen to the heartbeat! It sounds somewhat like something from a submarine movie, but that's *your child*!

The pelvic and vaginal exam generally come last. For this she is on her back, usually with her legs up in stirrups. A speculum is used to spread open the vagina. Both by sight and feel, the doctor can determine the condition of the external and internal parts. Using a sterile glove, the doctor can examine the condition of the vagina and of the cervix. Simultaneously the amount of space the baby will have to move down the birth canal between the pelvic bones can be determined. This lets the doctor know if there are likely to be problems during the birth.

If the coloration of the vagina has changed to a bluish-purple (Chadwick's sign), a woman is almost certain to be pregnant. The vagina will have also become more elastic.

The cervix may have already become sealed off by a mucus plug, depending on how soon the mother goes in. The cervix itself will have softened somewhat (after the eighth week), taking on the feel of flesh rather than the feel of cartilage. (In *Textbook for Midwives*, by Margaret R. Myles, the difference is described as comparing the lips to the tip of the nose.)

Size and condition of the uterus are determined. This is done by holding it between two fingers inserted into the vagina and then pushing down on the abdomen from above (Hegar's sign). Somewhere between the seventh and eighth weeks, the growth can be noticed by skilled touch. By the twelfth week the uterus has grown to about twice its non-pregnant size.

It's fairly routine for the doctor to do a *Pap smear* (the full name is Papanicolaou smear) at this time. Since the speculum is already in place, it's quick and simple to take a sample of internal tissues by using a spatula designed for the task. Tests can then be made to determine the presence of malignant and/or cancerous cells. (Many physicians recommend that the female have a Pap smear done every year or so, whether she is pregnant or not. It is also becoming more common to use a special camera to take a picture of the cervix, as a diagnostic tool.)

It's possible that various other tests will also be made. For example, a urinalysis is virtually always done, and is often repeated each time the mother visits the doctor. The urinalysis reveals excessive levels of glucose or protein. It's not unusual for a pregnant woman to become diabetic, especially if she is older and pregnant for the first time. (Many physicians will order additional tests for diabetes if Mom is older than thirty, and almost certainly if she is thirty-five or older.) This dangerous condition can usually be controlled, but it's important to detect it early.

Another test is for the presence of human chorionic gonadotropin (HCG) in the urine. This hormone is responsible for the inhibition of the menstrual cycle. The HCG level begins a climb within about a week of conception. It reaches a peak about two months after the last menstrual period, which is one reason why the woman is often told to wait a couple of months before going to see the doctor to determine pregnancy. If you suspect pregnancy, let it serve as a reminder of the importance of a well-balanced diet, and the possible need for changes in lifestyle. However, this is not the time for her to begin taking vitamin supplements. Not without a doctor's recommendation. Lack of the hormone (a negative test result) doesn't necessarily mean that the woman is not pregnant. An excess of this hormone can also indicate a cyst, particularly on the fallopian tubes.

Tests for HCG are done both with urine and, more accurately, with blood. These tests have been refined in recent years and can be used within just a few days of the missed menstrual period. Even home testing kits are available. Regardless, no reasonable and positive degree of accuracy can be expected until two weeks after the missed menstrual period (about four weeks after conception). A positive result even this early is often considered to be 90 percent accurate or better. A negative test result is considered to be almost meaningless.

Normally, none of the tests or exam indications can be considered *absolutely* positive until somewhere between the sixteenth and twentieth weeks. The earlier the exam, the more uncertain the findings. Prior to eight weeks (two months), the findings are often misleading.

Pregnancy isn't absolute and certain until the examiner detects fetal movement, fetal heartbeat, or, via X ray, a fetal skeleton. (If the doctor hears the heart of the fetus or feels it move, for example, the only possible conclusion is that there is a fetus in there.) This generally isn't possible until somewhere after the sixteenth week.

However, although any one indication can be explained by some other cause, the combination of signs and symptoms is generally considered conclusive. If the breasts are enlarging, the areola are darkening, Montgomery's tubercles are appearing, the vagina is becoming purple, her periods have greatly lessened or have ceased, the cervix is sealing and has softened—all of which will happen within the first couple of months—the examiner can be almost certain that the mother is pregnant. In fact, experienced obstetricians can usually be better than 90 percent certain within a matter of minutes, and better than 99 percent sure when the examination has been completed.

After the exam, chances are good that the doctor will order a glucose-tolerance test. A glucose drink will be given to Mom. After an hour, a blood sample will be taken and tested. The reason is to test for the tendency toward gestational diabetes. If the test shows this tendency, the test will probably be repeated right away, and depending on the results, may be repeated periodically during the pregnancy.

Other Tests

A number of tests might be ordered fairly quickly during the pregnancy. You don't need to worry much about them. If the doctor calls for them, they will almost always be explained thoroughly. If they are not, and even if they are, never hesitate to ask questions. Not only do you deserve to know, often the doctor may recognize potential problems merely by the open communication.

A common test is *ultrasound*. This can be performed anytime during the pregnancy, but is more likely during the later months. It's also used in conjunction with other tests. The purpose is to use sound to see inside. Although no test is completely risk-free, ultrasound is considered far safer than any other method. With it the doctor can detect a multiple birth, a difficult pregnancy, birth defects, and much more.

Amniocentesis involves inserting a needle through the abdomen and into the amniotic sac to get a sample of the fluid for testing. Ultrasound is used to help guide the needle. The usual purpose is to detect potential birth defects, particularly those caused by genetics and/or chromosome damage. If needed, this test is usually done between the fifteenth and eighteenth week, but could be called for at other times.

If this kind of test is needed earlier (to detect chromosomal abnormalities), the doctor may opt for a CVS—*chorionic villi sampling.* A thin tube is moved through the cervix to get a sample of the placenta. Most often this test will be done between weeks nine and eleven, but again, it might be ordered at another time in the pregnancy. It is considered slightly less accurate than an amniocentesis, and doubles the risk a miscarriage from 1 to 2 percent, but the results come back faster. (It should be noted that many experts say that the increase in risk is due to the circumstances that call for the test, not the test itself.)

If the amniocentesis shows reason for concern, *a precutaneous umbilical blood sampling* (PUBS) might be done. The needle used is finer and is inserted into the umbilical cord directly to get a sample of the blood. Results of the test are usually available within three days.

Other than ultrasound, which is sometimes used almost to give a thrill to the parents, these tests will generally be avoided unless there is a good reason for them. It's possible that the parents won't be informed of the results—usually because the parents have specifically requested to not be informed. (Ultrasound and other tests may also be used to determine other problems.)

False Pregnancy

The technical term for false pregnancy is *pseudocyesis*. This describes a condition in which the woman experiences all the signs and symptoms of pregnancy without being pregnant, and possibly without even having had intercourse. There are documented cases in which the woman is so convinced of being pregnant that the abdomen swells, and "at term" she even experiences labor pains. (There are also documented cases of men experiencing pseudocyesis, which goes far beyond the "sympathy pains" men very often experience, and often find themselves the brunt of jokes as a result.)

As with everything else, there are a variety of explanations for this relatively unusual condition. The couple, and especially the mother, might want the pregnancy so much that psychosomatic symptoms set in. At times these symptoms can be so strong that even an experienced doctor can be fooled.

Consider a woman who has desperately wanted a baby for a long time. She might miss her period due to stress. Stress can cause an increase in blood pressure, which in turn can stimulate a wide variety of other symptoms, including the purpling of the vagina. This in turn causes other things to happen, which can cause other things to happen, which in turn . . .

In short, Mom can fool herself into thinking that she is pregnant to such an extreme that she'll begin to show all the signs and symptoms. Only an expert can tell the difference, and even *they* can be fooled at times (until fetal heartbeat is heard, or not heard, for example). False pregnancy is rare, but it is possible.

Couvade Syndrome

Although it has never been seriously studied, indications are that at least 20 percent of all fathers experience the symptoms of pregnancy and labor. Obviously he's not pregnant, nor in labor, but this doesn't make the symptoms any less real. He can get morning sickness, sore back, swelling limbs, contractions, and more.

Just why this happens is unknown. It could be sympathetic in nature, be involved with stress, or have some other cause. In any case, it's nothing new. Medical writings from four hundred years ago mention it. In some cultures it is not only accepted, it becomes a part of the social customs.

Should you experience symptoms, don't be alarmed. It's not unusual. You should also be aware, however, that these symptoms can be caused by various ailments. Some of these are potentially quite serious. It might be a good idea to schedule a checkup for yourself. That way you'll be sure, and will have the benefit of knowing that you are in good health for what is to come.

The First Changes

As already mentioned, a number of changes will take place. The mother will miss a period, or will have a very light one. The breasts will tend to enlarge and to become more tender. The nipples tend to enlarge and darken. Later on the breasts may begin to secrete fluid, either spontaneously or after squeezing them.

Especially in the first few months, she may experience morning sickness. When she first gets up, there will be a queasiness and slight dizziness. This could lead to possible and occasional vomiting. Normally this is no problem. If it continues or is severe, get medical help. Her condition is probably fine, but there's no sense in taking chances.

As things progress, the *linea nigra* may begin to appear, running from the pubic region to the navel and possibly a little farther. (Note that this darkish line usually fades or disappears entirely after the birth.) The tummy might also begin to bulge slightly, although you have to look carefully in the first months. (Most women don't "show" until about twenty weeks.) More fathers feel an additional firmness, rather than see a difference, in the early stages.

A fairly rare but often frightening symptom is called the "mask of pregnancy." With this, parts of the body, usually the face, darken. The marks can be red, purple, and sometimes brown, and look much like a birthmark. In severe cases the marks can cover much of the neck and face. Even then, however, the marks will usually fade and disappear after the birth.

Perhaps more important to the baby's father, a woman could begin to experience mood shifts. One minute she might be cheerful and happy, and the next she might start crying or could even fly into a rage for no apparent reason. There's not much you can do for this other than to keep in mind that she probably can't help herself. Your job through this is to do your best to maintain an understanding of what is going on, and why.

If she has ever started taking oral contraceptives while you've known her, you may already be familiar with the mood swings that are possible. (The Pill basically makes the woman's body *think* it's pregnant to prevent actual pregnancy. It's not uncommon for a woman who is just starting to take oral contraceptives to exhibit mood swings until her body adjusts to the drug.)

Inside her body there are massive shifts in the hormonal and enzyme balance. Imagine yourself suddenly injected with a variety of mood-shifting drugs. If someone were doing that to you, you'd probably feel that your sudden and unpredictable shifts in mood were not your own fault. They wouldn't be. Well, Mom is going through that during pregnancy. Quite often she will feel guilty about screaming at you for no reason and will feel foolish for crying. The pregnancy itself is doing that. Her once familiar body is suddenly under the influence of something beyond her control.

Just how to handle that situation depends primarily on you and on her. Overcoddling can make matters worse, especially if she sees you as her source of strength. Screaming back can also make matters worse. Hopefully you know her well enough to be able to handle the situation. Your job as a loving spouse is to simply do your best to cope, and to forgive those temporary outbursts. They mean nothing, and are not the release of hidden hostilities.

Rest assured, those mood shifts almost never last long. If she has been screaming at you and there is honestly no reason for it, an hour or so later she might be cuddling under your arm. She might also have gone back to the bedroom to cry.

Relax. Try to maintain your normal lifestyle as best you can. At worst, the condition won't last forever. Probably the best advice is "Hang in there."

What's Coming?

The answer to this is simple but vague. A LOT is coming! Even if you've been through it before, there are going to be changes and surprises you can't even imagine. No two pregnancies are alike.

What's coming on a more mundane level will be something like the following.

The first visit to the doctor normally comes somewhere between two and three months after conception, although a first visit at four or even five months isn't uncommon. She will generally be asked to come back every three weeks up to the twenty-eighth week; then every two weeks up to the thirty-fourth week. In the last weeks, she'll probably be seeing the doctor every week.

Most of the visits will last less than ten minutes (unless there are any complications or there are a number of questions on her part or yours). Weight and blood pressure are taken each time. Almost always she'll provide a small amount of urine for testing.

The regular visits basically consist of recording her weight and blood pressure, the urine analysis, the doctor asking her if everything is okay and does she (or you) have any questions, listening to the baby, and doing an abdominal palpation and measurement. Toward the end the doctor will probably also do a pelvic and vaginal exam to keep a close track of the condition of the cervix and birth canal as "her time" approaches, and to help to more accurately determine just when that "time" will be.

Mom is going to go through changes that you may have never experienced. These will be physical and emotional. She'll probably be concerned that she is "blowing up like a whale." She is likely to have a variety of fears, from the fear that you don't love her anymore, to the fear of a deformed child, to the fear of the pain, to other fears she sometimes can't even name. Keep in mind that this is all happening at a time when her body is being flooded with new levels of hormones and enzymes. She may often feel out of control.

She might worry about everything she does, or doesn't do. At times she might seem to be almost obsessed with health, diet, exercise, the home, and basically everything around her. A tiny muscle spasm could throw her into a panic. She could blame you for "forcing" her into having a glass of wine to celebrate the news about the pregnancy.

More than a few fathers report that they feel out of control themselves. They might find themselves suddenly and inexplicably slamming doors and screaming about a tiny spot on the kitchen floor. Or, for no reason they can name, all of a sudden Mom seems sexier and more desirable than ever before, but this gets coupled with a fear of injuring her or the child. Men often feel a stronger sense of protectiveness.

For all this, your job is a difficult one. On one hand, you need to provide love, support, understanding, and cool-headedness. On the other, don't pretend to be a doctor. Some of her fears just might be legitimate. It could be a tough judgment call. It might help you to know that this reaction in her is not only normal but is often considered to be desirable. It shows that she is developing a strong sense of responsibility for the life inside her.

Then there are your own fears. These might be financial, feelings of inadequacy, fears of losing your wife's affections, not knowing how to change a diaper. . . . You might find yourself regretting that you participated in making her pregnant, even if it was planned. You might even find yourself wondering at times if this woman is *really* the one you want to mother your children.

As with almost everything else in the world, it is a two-way street. Often both sides will claim that the other has no idea what they are going through. That's a very true and valid claim. Like it or not, no matter how you try, you can't know what your mate is experiencing. You can gather as much information as possible and make a good guess. You can imagine. How can a father ever understand completely what a pregnant woman is feeling? He can't.

At the same time, and just as valid, how can the woman understand completely what the "pregnant" father is experiencing? She can't.

Both are realities you have to face early. Both of you are going to be experiencing more changes than you might realize. You as the father are not the focus of attention, she is. At times you'll feel left out, as though those around you, including your mate, don't want anything to do with you, and don't consider you important. "You provided the sperm. Your job is done. Now get out of the way."

This is one of the things you're just going to have to face, just as Mom will be facing morning sickness and swollen legs and the pain of giving birth.

It's a hard time. It's also a great time. The major difference is in your own attitude.

What Can You Do?

This is another question easily answered, but with a useless answer. "Not much. And everything." Ambiguous but very true. This might be your tenth child, but if it is, you'll already know that no two pregnancies are alike. If she was affectionate and considerate last time, that doesn't mean that you won't find breakfast cereal in your lap this time. If she had the tendency to lock you out of the bedroom with the last child, you might feel like you're on a nine-month-long honeymoon this time around. Or there might be no appreciable changes in your home life at all. Unfortunately, there's no way to predict it.

It's not easy to remain calm, loving, and understanding when your normally lovely lady is screaming at you for no reason, or starts crying, also for no reason. (Or at least no reason you know about. She probably doesn't know, either.)

Be aware some of the things that seem senseless to you might be very important to her. This is a time when you have to use your own best judgment. You know her. When the hormonal shifts kick into gear, you might even know her better than she knows herself. Will she benefit most if you just simply get out of the way for a while? If so, get out of the way. Maybe she's one of those who needs you to tell her, "Stop it!" Keep in mind that something that worked well yesterday could worsen the same situation tomorrow.

More important is what you do afterward. If she has just screamed at you, then comes to you for a hug, let your anger go! Keep in mind that she can't help it, and that she probably feels as bad about it, or worse, than you do. If you're angry or upset, go outside and dig a hole or pound some nails or run around the block. Not only will you work off the anger, the exercise will do you good and may even help to get you in shape for the long labor that is coming. (Her job at that time will certainly be more strenuous, but don't fall for the false notion that labor is hard only on the woman. It's not unusual for the father to come out of the delivery room every bit as exhausted as the mother.)

Throughout the pregnancy, your moral and physical support is important. A little pampering can go a long way at this time. It will make things easier on Mom, which in turn will make things easier on you, and on your relationship. The two of you will come closer together. The environment of love and friendship will extend to the birth itself, making that easier, and making the recovery easier.

Think of it another way. Pregnancy is *not* a sickness, but for just a moment think of it as one. Now compare two people who are sick. One of them gets no support and no care. When a fever causes this person to say something she doesn't mean, those around her yell back and leave. In the second case, the person is cared for and made to feel important. A few flare-ups here and there are forgiven and (just as important) forgotten.

Which "patient" will be better off?

It has been shown that a mother who feels lost and afraid will have a much worse pregnancy. The pregnancy is more complicated. So is the birthing. More goes wrong. From the doctor's perspective, there are more lawsuits.

This is one of the primary driving forces behind getting the father involved. Of course, it's better and more fulfilling for the father. As important as this is, it's still secondary. Never forget that the mother and child MUST come first. When Mom has her loved one(s) at her side and giving her constant support, everything tends to be smoother. This can literally prevent many problems from happening in the first place, will reduce the seriousness of them, and will greatly reduce any risks.

There's no way to accurately predict what is going to happen, or when. In most cases her normal personality will remain, and any mood shifts tend to be temporary and short-lived. The same is true of the various physical problems. The sore back, the swollen feet, and all the other symptoms will disappear. It may take a little work, but her body can return to how it was before the pregnancy, or very nearly so.

In short, pregnancy is a temporary condition. The more you take part, the more you can enjoy the experience. The more you learn and know, the better you'll be able to control the situation for both you and your loved (and soon-to-be-loved) ones.

There will be sacrifices to be made. If you think of them as sacrifices, they'll be more difficult. If you think of them as one more way to become an integral part, that's just what they'll become. The difference is in your attitude.

Meanwhile, when you find that Mom is going to be Mom (and you are going to be DADDY!), you probably have about seven months, tops, before the baby will come into the world and into your life. That may seem like a long time, but it shoots by fast. The sooner you start your preparations, the better.

There are a lot of things to be done.

3

Doctors, Hospitals, and Alternatives

*I*magine an extreme case. Your wife is in labor. You're lost and unable to find the hospital. You've already had to stop to get gas because the tank was almost dry. ("I'll get it on the way to work in the morning," you'd told yourself.) Finally, with the help of a policeman, you arrive. He wheels your wife into Admitting while you try to figure out just where the parking lot is located. Then you end up sitting in the waiting room while the red tape of registration is handled, a detail made more difficult because you can't remember the name of the doctor. Your wife knows but has already been taken to the labor and delivery room. Now off you go in another direction to arrange the financial matters.

While you're trying to remember your mother-in-law's maiden name for the paperwork, you're already a father. Mom is extremely tired and in a poor state of mind for making important decisions, and you're not there to help. The nurse wants to know what name to put on the birth certificate at a time when Mom is lucky to know her own name. But you're not there. You're still downstairs filling out papers and the check.

You've missed the birth. Both of you have shredded nerves, which has ruined the joy you might have shared, and the confusion has even made giving birth more difficult for your wife.

At long last you get home again, but there's no place to put the baby. You don't have a crib. You don't even have suitable blankets or clothing. There are no diapers. No baby supplies at all, and nothing the new mother needs. Just when your presence is most needed at home, you find yourself running around like mad trying to find and buy all the things you need, with little idea of just what that is. Making it worse yet, you're expected to show up at work promptly at 7:30 A.M. the next morning.

That's no way to enjoy your new baby.

The solution is to be prepared well ahead of time. As many of the decisions as possible should have already been made before labor begins. For those that can't be made ahead of time, at least anticipate what might happen, what your options are, and how you (both of you) intend to handle it.

How much you leave to the last minute determines how well the birthing will work for you, your wife, and the baby. Trying to squeeze months of decisions and details into a couple of days is an invitation for disaster, and almost a guarantee that you won't be able to enjoy things as much as you could. Leaving all those details until the birthing is in progress is worse yet.

This carries through into preparing the home, but begins by selecting the doctor(s) and hospital, and taking care of the details and finances.

The Doctor

The following assumes that your wife doesn't already have her own doctor, or rather doesn't have a doctor who can deliver babies. If she does, "choosing a doctor" becomes irrelevant, because you already have one.

You probably won't be playing much of a part in choosing a doctor. The actual choice has to be made by your mate. *She* is the patient and the one dealing directly with the doctor, and *she* is the one to make the decision. This doesn't mean that you shouldn't become involved in making the choice. The choice will be hers, but your own input can be valuable. Or it might be useless and even unwanted. That should be fine, too.

A number of people pick their doctor by paging through the phone book and finding the one who is closest. Others choose their doctor based on a recommendation from a friend or other family member. Both methods are okay, and both have disadvantages.

In the first case, location means very little other than convenience, and possibly a link between the doctor(s) and the nearest hospital. It says nothing about competence or ability. Convenience is certainly a factor, but is no indicator of competence.

Recommendations from friends and family may or may not be meaningful. It depends a lot on how well they know that doctor and what that doctor has done for them. Imagine a close friend who has highly recommended Dr. Smith. This doctor has done wonders for your friend's hernia, but can that same doctor also expertly deliver a child and handle complications?

Even if the recommended doctor is an ob-gyn and handles births as a daily routine, that doesn't necessarily mean that he or she is the doctor the two of you want to deliver your own child.

If you have a family doctor who takes care of other matters (your own doctor, for example, or better yet, her regular doctor), you have a built-in source for a recommendation. All you have to do is ask. If you're not comfortable calling to ask just that question, maybe it's time for you to have a physical. It sure can't hurt to know that you're in tip-top shape, and simultaneously you'll have the chance to ask for his recommendation at the same time. (Note that you should do this only with your wife's knowledge and permission.)

If you think that you have absolutely no sources at all, don't give up. You can once again take care of several things at one time by calling local hospitals to inquire about childbirth classes. This will give you the chance to check out the hospital, to check out the childbirth classes, and to get a recommendation from the class instructor—someone who again deals with this sort of thing every day.

The age of the doctor is often used as a basis for the choice. This may or may not be valid. It's a fair rule of thumb that a doctor who has been around longer will have the valuable (possibly crucial!) experience and will have successfully handled more emergencies and difficulties. However, the older doctor is also more likely to be set in his ways. More important, age is no guarantee of competence.

The younger doctor obviously has less practical experience, but might be more up-to-date on the newest techniques. Also remember that even the newest doctor has had years of intense training and experience just to become licensed.

Also important is the doctor's attitude. Does he truly put the mother and child first? What is his attitude toward you and your participation?

That last works in both directions. Some doctors (not many these days) don't want the father involved at all. Others go in the opposite direction. One new father found out the hard way just how much their doctor wanted him involved. As the baby was being born, the doctor called the father down and said, "Get ready to catch the baby. Here it comes." Then he stepped back, leaving the bewildered father to ease his child from the womb.

While there are few things quite like "catching" your baby, the doctor merely assumed that the father would do it, and the father assumed he'd be holding his wife's hand at the other end of the birthing table.

A Female Physician?

Throughout this book the doctor, and certain other professionals involved, are usually referred to as "he." This is done merely to ease the reading. (Having to constantly read "he or she" and "him or her" can become ponderous.) This is certainly no indication that there aren't some truly wonderful women doctors. Gender has nothing to do with intelligence or competence.

The reality is that medicine, including obstetrics, has been dominated by males for a very long time. There are more male doctors than female (and more female nurses than male). Whatever your feelings about it, this is how things are.

Today, at least in obstetrics, the proportion of males to females is reversing. Soon there will be as many, and perhaps more, female obstetricians than male. The female obstetrician, at least those who have been pregnant, have a distinct advantage. It's true that no two pregnancies are alike, but someone who has at least gone through it is likely to have some insights that aren't available to someone (male or female) who hasn't.

Ideally the choice will be made solely on ability, competence, and experience. Realistically, personal views sometimes make gender an issue. Your job as the father is to make sure that *you* aren't the one who makes it an issue.

Some women prefer to have another woman as the obstetrician. This is "her time." Her level of comfort is all-important. If she prefers a female doctor and you find yourself not liking the idea, swallow those feelings and let it go. At the same time, if you find yourself feeling uncomfortable at having another man examine your wife and *you* want her to see a female doctor, while she doesn't want this, once again you must swallow those feelings. It's truly none of your business.

So relax, and always put your wife's comfort, and safety, first.

Group Practices

More and more doctors, especially obstetricians, are going into group practice. They'll often have one or two partners, and sometimes more. The reason for this should be obvious.

Think of the obstetrician's schedule. One in solo practice is on call twenty-four hours a day, 365 days a year (or 366). He'll see patients all day long, but will have no guarantee at all of being able to relax once he gets home, or even be able to sleep through the night. In short, he's under a lot of pressure and is almost always in a rush. Further, if he's already at the birth of another of his patients or is otherwise not available, your baby will be delivered by whoever happens to be on call at the hospital at that time.

With a group practice, the partners share in the responsibilities. Most likely, during the pregnancy each of the partners will see the mother on a rotating basis so that each of them has at least some familiarity with the case. Whichever of them happens to be on call at the time will deliver the baby. That one may not be your favorite, but at least it will be someone both of you know, and more important, someone who is familiar with your wife.

A disadvantage is that the attention is spread across several doctors. Most likely your wife will "officially" have only one doctor responsible for her. The partners fill in when the primary doctor isn't available, or, as above, on a rotating basis to become at least a little familiar with each other's patients.

The Hospital and Its Policies

Often the doctor you choose will dictate the hospital you'll be using. Most doctors have privileges at just so many local hospitals, sometimes at only one. In reverse, the hospital you prefer might dictate the doctor you have.

Assuming that you'll be having the baby in a hospital (almost 99 percent of all people do), the choice of doctor and hospital go hand in hand. They work together. If the doctor you and your wife choose isn't allied with the hospital you want, you'll either have to change hospitals or change doctors.

The regulations and attitudes of the hospital are every bit as important as those of the doctor. Perhaps more so. Some hospitals are advanced enough that they go well out of their way to encourage the father to participate as fully as possible, and leave any restrictions to the doctor. A few have such strict policies that even the most open-minded doctor won't be able to get the father past the waiting room. (These days, this is extremely rare.) Most hospitals are somewhere between. What's important is that you find out ahead of time.

You can expect to come across some restrictions no matter where you go. In most cases there are good reasons for those to be a part of hospital policy. Some exist for the convenience of the hospital and staff. True. The majority are in place so that the patients get the best possible care.

Sometimes the husband, siblings, and the newborn's grandparents are allowed to visit anytime, and can even stay twenty-four hours a day if they wish. Typically other relatives and friends can come in during generous visiting hours, but can be in the room only when the newborn is not.

This last might seem restrictive, but there is some sense behind it, especially since the regulation usually allows exceptions. (For example, if the mother's birthing coach was an unrelated close friend, that friend usually receives all the privileges of the father.) By restricting visitation, infection of the newborn, at least while under the care and responsibility of the hospital, is kept at a minimum, while still allowing unrestricted visitation by those who matter most. Other visitors can still see the newborn through a viewing window, and at worst may have to wait a day or two to hold the child once the parents have gone home.

By most hospital regulations, if anesthesia, such as for a C-section, becomes necessary, or any emergency at all comes up, the father might be asked to leave the room. (He will probably be allowed to attend the C-section operation, assuming the doctor allows it.) This is fairly common, and again there is some sense behind it. The time needed to prep the mother for surgery also gives the father time to prepare to enter the operating area. A sterile field is critical in such cases. Also is the fact that many laypersons panic at such times and can get in the way.

However, there are still policies that do make little sense. Despite encouraging fathers to stay it's not unusual for there to be no facilities made available for the father. If he is hungry, he has to leave the room, and sometimes the hospital. He may not be offered so much as a glass of water or cup of coffee, unless the mother orders it for herself and gives it to him.

In other words, the husband can stay twenty-four hours a day, assuming he doesn't need food, water, or a place to sleep, and doesn't mind going without a shower or bath for a few days.

Such a condition can be tolerated, assuming that all other more important factors stand true. This may not even be of importance to you personally. If your intention is to be there for the birthing and then go home, then off to work or whatever, the lack of sleeping arrangements or dinner won't matter. Even if you intend to be there around the clock until Mom and the baby come home, sleeping in a chair one or two nights isn't an insurmountable problem.

Still, with a bit of searching and researching, and possibly some ahead-of-time arrangements, you may not even have to tolerate the inconvenience. Set your own standards. Find what minimums you can accept, while remembering to *always* put the needs of the mother and child first.

Choosing the Hospital

First priority is medical competence and complete medical facilities. Some hospitals can handle only routine birthings. (Some aren't set up to handle birthings at all.) Others can handle Level 2 (minor complications) or even Level 3 (complications including life-threatening ones). At very least, the hospital you use should have access, preferably by helicopter, to the higher-level facilities should that become necessary. It probably won't, but preparation for those rare eventualities can make a life-or-death difference.

Of secondary concern, but still of great importance, is how the hospital feels about the mother, her rights, and the rights of the infant. Most hospitals have given in to the pressure of good common sense. They treat the mother and infant with due respect and attention to their needs. The days of routinely drugging the mother heavily, even "for her own good," are gone. A few hospitals still remain, however, that routinely separate the mother and child immediately after

birth, and don't put them together again until it is convenient for the hospital.

Note that this doesn't include those hospitals that separate the mother and child for medical reasons. That kind of
thing shows that the hospital is concerned, responsible, and
competent. If there is a medical reason for the separation,
the hospital is doing the job it's supposed to, namely that of
putting the welfare of the mother and child first.

Typically, immediately after the birth the baby is taken
aside to be cleaned and given a quick examination. After the
attending staff determines that the child is healthy, it is returned to the mother. She may or may not be instructed how
to breast-feed the child, depending on the circumstances and
the wishes of the mother. In almost every case, the parents
are not rushed but are given time to enjoy being new parents.

Eventually Mom will be taken to a recovery room. (Becoming more and more popular is the LDR room. Labor, delivery, and recovery happen in one place. Mom isn't moved
until she is in "recuperation.") The baby is taken to a nursery. This gives Mom a chance to rest, and the staff to examine
the baby more thoroughly. Normally, unless there is a definite reason to deny it, all Mom has to do is ask and the baby
will be brought to her, and left for as long as she wishes.

If a major emergency occurs, you can expect to be asked
to leave at least temporarily, but what if the situation calls
for a C-section? This is normal procedure, as explained
above. More important is, how do the doctor and hospital
feel about C-section births in general? How often are they
done? This is both an indication and a *possible* warning. The
doctor should be skilled and experienced enough to perform
one if it becomes necessary, but shouldn't be *too* willing or
quick to exercise that option. Likewise, the hospital policy
shouldn't be one that encourages performing this operation
(such as for time constraints).

It will be hard for you to tell whether a C-section is actually required. You aren't a medical expert, and this is the

kind of decision that requires that expertise. This is the job of the doctor, and he should be able to make it for valid cause, not just because the hospital policy encourages a C-section if labor goes beyond a certain number of hours.

To be fair, although there are some who claim that many hospitals (and doctors) have such policies, and even that some hospitals encourage C-sections for higher profits, it's unlikely that this is common. At least not for those reasons.

Ideally the hospital will allow rooming in. This means that the baby can be with the mother as much as the mother wishes (dependent, of course, on the physical condition of the mother and the baby). A hospital with such a policy has recognized the importance of the mother/child relationship. Almost without fail, that hospital will also offer whatever assistance and teaching the mother needs to breast-feed and care for the baby in any way.

It never hurts to ask. Find out everything you can about anything and everything that is of concern to you. Do so well ahead of time! In fact, you'll probably find that the hospital gives guided tours of the birthing center.

Attitudes

All through the pregnancy and birth, and even after, you're likely to be facing the attitudes of others involved, and of those not involved. Much of this you can simply ignore. For example, you're bound to run across a few people who have the idea that once the man "plants his seed," the only thing he should do is write the checks and stay out of the way. As one feminist publication put it, "Pregnancy and childbirth is thoroughly feminine. Men have no business even *thinking* about being involved." (This same publication stated, "The average father spends just fourteen seconds per week with his children." That is so obviously false that it is equally obvious that the author has a serious attitude problem.)

Attitudes as severe as this are fortunately rare. However, you can almost count on running into some milder versions of it. Most of these will be merely irritating and can be (should be!) ignored. As long as this comes from the outside and isn't affecting or interfering with your right as a father to be involved with your wife, the pregnancy, and your child, don't be concerned.

Far more important is when those attitudes do cause an effect, especially when the person holding the attitudes is in a position of authority. For example, how does the doctor feel about your participation? How about the hospital? The nursing staff? Are you accepted, or just barely tolerated?

Some doctors and nurses still seem to have the attitude that Dad is relatively unimportant—that you're in the way. (Be aware that sometimes this is true.) Keep in mind at all times, despite background, credentials, and importance, they are still *your* employees. You're paying *them*, not the other way around. Unless you are truly interfering, they have no right or business to exclude or ignore you.

At the same time, remember *why* they are your employees. They are the experts. You've hired them for their knowledge, skills, and experience. Listen. Don't accept blindly, but listen.

Be honest and straightforward with the doctor, and he's likely to answer in kind. If you find that he's just not right for you, he can probably recommend someone who is, and will probably be very willing to do so. (However, once again keep in mind that the choice of doctor is *Mom's* decision, not yours. You're in this to help, not to control.)

Hospital attitudes—actually hospital *policies*—may not be subject to as much discussion. Most of these won't affect you as much as you might think. It's common for the hospital to welcome a participating father, and rare for a hospital to deny him unless there is a very good reason for it.

When It's Not Right

One mistake that many people make is to forget that they have the right to find another doctor, or another hospital, if they think that they can do better elsewhere. If the two of you pick the doctor who *seems* to be right for you only to find out that some of his ways of doing things aren't in agreement with what you want, don't hesitate. Find someone else.

You've hired him for his expertise, but *you* and (more important) your wife are the boss. If your "employee" isn't doing things as you want, "fire" him. That may sound harsh, but think about it. This is one of the most important events in your lives. A child is to be born. *Your* child. Besides, no doctor wants an unwilling patient.

If there is a conflict, first talk to the doctor. The whole problem may simply be a lack of communication. He may not realize that a conflict exists and will be willing to adapt to take care of it (assuming that the objection is realistic).

Payments

One couple lived in a rural area thirty miles from the hospital. Another was within walking distance. Both women went into the first stages of labor on a Tuesday afternoon. Tuesday night around 10:00 P.M. the first woman was taking a shower because she wanted to feel clean for the birthing. The second was sitting in a waiting room at the hospital while her husband began filling out papers. At midnight the first couple parked, came inside, gave their names, and in about two minutes were off to a room that was waiting for them. The second couple was still in the lobby.

A part of this was lack of preparation in general. The first woman had a regular doctor whom she'd been seeing for months. When she went into labor, the first and most obvious call went to the doctor. The symptoms, plus the awareness and mutual participation between doctor and parents, had the doctor calling the hospital. When the couple arrived, the room was ready. The only thing left was to sign the admission papers. These were also ready, needing only the signature. All the basic costs, calculated and based on the regular examinations, had been prepaid.

The second couple didn't have a doctor, hadn't taken care of any arrangements . . . and, because it wasn't an emergency, were confined to sitting in the waiting room while paperwork was being filled out and credit references checked.

Face a hard reality. Very few things in life are free. Once you have your doctor and hospital, you'll have something else. Bills. The doctor has to be paid. So does the hospital. Quite often a payment schedule is set up so that most or all of the fees are paid before the due date. Stick to that schedule—or beat it. Getting behind not only strains the doctor/patient relationship, it can be deadly to your checking account balance. If $125 is owed this month, and $125 next, but you miss this month, next month you'll owe $250, then $375, then $500. It adds up fast, and as it does, it becomes more and more difficult to pay, especially when you're also trying to buy baby furniture and supplies, and are also trying to prepay the hospital.

If you simply cannot afford to make a payment, don't get embarrassed and lie about it to the doctor. "Oh, I forgot to bring my checkbook." Be honest about it. Arrangements can almost always be made. Besides, if you can trust the doctor with the lives and well-being of your wife and child, can't you trust him with something of relatively little importance, such as a temporary (hopefully) financial shortage?

Do everything possible to plan ahead financially. Ideally all fees should be paid in full at least a month before the child is due to be born. Preferably earlier. All the needed paperwork, including admission forms, should also be filled out.

The exact costs will vary widely, depending on a number of factors. Rates vary in different parts of the country. It's not unusual for the rates to vary from hospital to hospital, and from doctor to doctor. If you choose an alternate method, such as a birthing center, all this is even more true. Any problems or complications will add to the cost. A C-section, for example, can easily add two thousand to five thousand dollars or more.

The key is to find out ahead of time. Most hospitals, birthing centers, and physicians have set "package rates." Do not be embarrassed about asking. This is not like shopping for a new car, but you have the right to know, and the right to compare.

Alternative Methods

Worldwide, approximately two thirds of all births are handled by midwives or their equivalent. Even in this country, the number of births handled by midwives went up nearly sevenfold in the 1970s (from about 20,000 to nearly 140,000). This trend has continued since then (although not at the same rate of increase). The idea that only the poor use a midwife because they are unable to afford "anything better" is quickly fading.

While there are still "granny" midwives around, the majority are C.N.M.s—certified nurse midwives. These people (almost invariably women) are registered nurses with a degree, who have also gone through extensive special training in giving birth. Quite often they are allied with local formal medical facilities, including obstetricians and obstetrical teams. More than a few work from a birthing center, which makes it possible for the mother to have her child in a very homelike atmosphere and with highly personal attention.

In general, C.N.M.s handle only low-risk clients. Careful screening makes sure that their clients are unlikely to have complications. When complications seem likely, the client is referred back to an obstetrician who is (possibly) better trained, and who is legally allowed to handle those emergencies.

The obstetrician is a busy person. Almost always he shows up at the last minute, delivers the baby, takes care of any surgical "patch-up" on Mom, and disappears again. No fault can be attached to this. It's necessary, due to the number of patients. (It's also important to realize that the doctor is quite willing, and able, to spend whatever time is needed. If his skills are needed for only an hour, there's no reason for him to hang around for six hours. If six hours are needed, he won't abandon the mother.)

The midwife often makes it a point to arrive at the hospital just about the same time that Mom does. She then stays with Mom through the labor and birth, leaving the room only when someone else who is qualified is standing by.

The advantage of a birthing center is that the mother (and you) is in control. Mom is the boss. There are rules and restrictions, as there must be, but they are not hard, fast, and inflexible. Nor is the father automatically excluded. The whole idea of the center is to provide a family atmosphere, and to bring control and dignity and joy to the birth.

Statistically, a first-time mother giving birth in a hospital, with the often less personal attention and automatic restrictions and regulations, tends to have a labor lasting between twelve and twenty-four hours. The incidence of infection— maternal and infant—is considerably higher in a hospital than in a birthing center, simply due to the fact that there are more sick people around. It's not all that unusual for someone to pick up a staph infection while in the hospital, and particularly while in an operating room.

Many birthing centers cite statistics that show a near zero

infection rate, and an average labor time for a first birth in the range of six hours.

The disadvantage is that the center isn't as capable of handling real emergencies as would be a hospital. They realize this, which is why they turn down clients who are at risk. It's very important that the to-be-parents are open and honest with the center. For example, if the mother has a history of spontaneous abortions and does not tell the attending midwife, unforeseen complications can arise that can put the lives of the mother and baby in danger.

Midwives and birthing centers point out that their success rate is considerably higher than that of hospitals. The infant mortality rate, the amount of time for maternal recovery, and the general physical condition of both mother and infant are very often better with a birthing center. This is a valid claim, but once again it must be noted that such centers accept only low-risk (or no-risk) patients. Hospitals accept, and are geared for, the more difficult cases. They are bound to have a somewhat lower success rate.

Some midwives encourage, under certain circumstances, birth at home. The idea is that this is where the mother is most comfortable and relaxed. Studies have shown that the mother's attitude plays a very large role in the birth. For some women, being at home and in familiar surroundings can make a great difference. For others, the surroundings are *too* familiar. They feel uncomfortable and even fearful without emergency medical equipment right on hand.

The disadvantages of using a birth center are magnified with a home birth. It is often suggested that couples who live a distance from a hospital not even consider a home birth. If serious complications arise during the birth, there simply may not be time to get to the hospital for professional care. The only equipment available is whatever the midwife brings along.

For either alternative, you have to be realistic.

The first and most important factor, as always, is the

health and safety of the mother and infant. If there are health problems that could cause a high-risk pregnancy, it's unrealistic and selfish to stick to the idea of having the baby at home. If mother and child are healthy and she has no history of difficulties, she *might* be a candidate for an alternative method. If she is unhealthy, drug-dependent, has a history of health and birth problems, if it is a multiple birth, if the fetal presentation is breech, or any of a number of other circumstances exist, giving birth in a hospital where emergency equipment and highly skilled people are immediately at hand is essential.

Second is how the mother feels about it. If she feels more comfortable and at ease in a hospital, that should be the end of the discussion. Her needs and desires MUST take precedence. In such a case, when a birthing center or home birth will make her more nervous and tense, you're defeating the main purpose of that alternative.

Keep in mind, this isn't a game. At least two lives are at stake. While you and your wife might find appealing the idea of having the baby in your own bedroom at home, don't do so simply because it's the "in thing" to do. This is a very serious decision that requires careful and honest examination.

At the same time, the use of a birthing center might be the perfect solution in your case. Don't go into it blindly, but don't close your mind to it as an option.

Childbirth Classes

An increasing number of hospitals are offering childbirth classes. Most charge a nominal fee (thirty-five dollars or so). Some are free. It's a fair bet that any hospital that is going to welcome the father will have such classes.

The reverse is also an indicator. If the hospital doesn't have such classes, it may not be set up to allow Dad to participate. (For that matter, the hospital might be one of the few remaining that doesn't even want Mom to participate.) If the hospital does not offer classes, it's time to find out for sure if you'll be allowed in the room, or if you should find another hospital.

Some class instructors are perhaps too used to the women knowing more than the men. To lighten the mood, humor is injected. You might find that this is done at the expense of the males present. If you come across this, ignore it. It's really not the standard, and certainly isn't important. *Mom* is important. The *child* is important. The *class* is important. An instructor's poor choice of humor should never stand in the way.

Place your concern where it needs to be, namely in gaining knowledge of what birthing is all about. This is the single greatest advantage of having gone through the childbirth classes.

Mom's tummy is getting bigger by the day. The baby is coming, and it's too late to change your minds now. You're *going* to have a baby. Like it or not, scared or not, that baby is coming. Plain and simple. Attending class helps to set that into your mind. Those classes get the two of you working in the same direction. Together. If you forget everything else that you learned in class, the working together will carry you through.

A close second is the knowledge about birthing. (That's why I wrote this book. And why you bought it!) Knowing what is coming can go a long, long way in helping to get you through it. The classes should teach both of you what is coming, and when it comes, you'll have at least some idea of what to expect.

For example, when there's a gush of water coming from the birth tract, you'll know that the amniotic sac has burst. Mom isn't dying. The blood that accompanies that gush, and the blood that comes both before and after, are probably normal (but it's still time to head for the hospital immediately!).

When the baby comes out with a distorted head, you'll know that you don't have a monster—just a normal baby that has been pushed through a narrow channel and with a skull that has soft spots to allow this. Everything is probably normal and just fine.

Chances are good that neither of you—and especially you—previously knew a whole lot about it. Childbirth classes attempt to teach you the basics in just a few short weeks.

Many fears can be set aside. This is important for you. It's particularly important for the mother. With you attending class right by her side, it is all made easier for her—something that extends into and through the actual birth, and beyond.

Both of you have undoubtedly heard many of the horror stories of giving birth. It's bad enough for you, since you're the one who has to sit back and let her go through those horrors, with nothing you can really do about it. Put yourself in her place. You have to stand by. *She* has to go through it. You could argue validly that either is worse than the other—but this isn't a contest.

Fears create problems—sometimes serious ones. That fact is one of the main driving forces behind prepared childbirth. The more Mom knows about what is *really* coming (as opposed to exaggerated horror stories), the fewer fears she will have, and the better she will be able to handle the situation.

This is primary. Mom *always* comes first.

What is often forgotten by the educators is that Dad is in there, too. Dad has fears all his own. The childbirth educators too often forget this simple fact because they're concentrating so much on Mom. (One of my hopes in writing this book is that more childbirth educators will come to realize this and address it in class as a valid and important topic.) Be prepared to have your own needs and fears ignored.

Yet another value of childbirth classes is learning the more specific relaxation techniques. Mom needs to learn to work *with* the contractions instead of resisting them.

Breathing helps considerably. Other techniques (conscious relaxation, and conscious flexing) tie in nicely. It's true that Mom will be the one doing it. It's just as true that having someone there to help, to coach, to remind and to guide, makes all of it so much easier. That's one of your jobs.

You can read books on these techniques, but that's of limited help. Actually seeing them demonstrated, then trying them, then having the instructor show how to do them better, is what will truly "bring them home."

That part of it is important, too. Bring them home. Practice together, as the instructor in class will almost certainly recommend.

No matter how you look at it, childbirth classes are very important. So go! Attend. Don't miss any sessions. And pay attention. Take notes. Make sketches in your notebook. Ask questions. Make the best use of this opportunity as possible.

If you already have children, and have been through this before, you might think that attending the class (or reading this book) has little value. Not true! Even if you have six children, each pregnancy is different. If nothing else, think of it as a refresher course, and as a means of regaining focus.

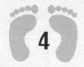

4

Other Preparations

*A*s mentioned in the last chapter, leaving all the decisions to the last minute is an invitation to disaster. There's no such thing as being *too* prepared. You have a lot to do over the next few months. More than you might realize. Once the baby is home, things will only become more hectic. The problem that many run into is in not planning ahead and being prepared.

Preparation isn't as complicated as you might think. Mostly what you're after is to get things set so that you can get through the birthing and through the first week or two afterward. Don't worry about six months, or six years, down the road.

Yet.

Choosing a Name

The time to talk about names for your child is well before you go to the hospital, not after the child is born. The hospital is going to want a name for the birth certificate fairly quickly. You, and especially your wife, will be tired. It's not the ideal time to be making decisions if you can help it. Choosing a name is actually one of the more important decisions the two of you will be making.

Imagine going through life as Ronald McDonald. Or as Harold (nicknamed Harry) Leggs. There are plenty of baby name books, complete with their origins and meanings. Take some time to go through them. Together. Not only will this help you find a name that is suitable and well thought out, discussing it can be fun.

Often it helps to write down the names. This gives you a way to actually see it in print and also serves as a good aid for discussion. Scratch out the rejected names. Keep the ones you've agreed upon. Then let those sit for a while. A week later a name that both of you loved may seem silly.

Take your time. If you start soon enough in the pregnancy, you'll have plenty of time to select names, reject them, select some new ones, maybe reselect ones you've turned down. Remember that this is the time to be changing your minds. Once the name is on the birth certificate, it's pretty much too late.

Circumcision

This can be a controversial subject, or nothing at all. Obviously, if the child is a girl, you don't have to worry. The discussion can also be closed (or never started) if your religious convictions make the decision for you.

Many people make the decision to circumcise the male baby on the basis that this is what most people do. Others absolutely refuse the procedure because of "modern" ideas (and even because of opinions espoused on talk-show programs).

There is no easy answer. At this time there is no conclusive evidence either way, for or against. It's a case in which for every pro there is a con, and vice versa.

As is so often the case, beware of the extremes. Perhaps a good example is the opinion that circumcision causes a lifelong psychological scar. It's possible (distantly) that a few newborns a day or two old might remember it, but ask one hundred circumcised males. Most will probably think the question is silly. They won't remember a thing about it.

If you are one of the many faced with the decision, first think about the operation itself.

The newborn is strapped to a small table. This prevents movement. The classic method is to use a scalpel to slice the foreskin of the penis. It is now more common to use a bell-shaped device that crushes the foreskin. Either way, there is very little blood.

The baby almost invariably cries out. Extreme proponents of circumcision say that the baby is crying from the frustration of being held immobile. At the opposite end, the picture is of a newborn screaming from torture. As usual, the truth is somewhere between.

Anesthetic is rarely used. The potential risks of anesthesia on the newborn's system could be considerable, and are often unpredictable. At the same time, being cut is painful. That pain will be forgotten, but the operation is bound to hurt. Despite the claims of some about the lifelong trauma—despite the claims of those who say it's really nothing—the truth is that we just don't know for certain.

There are cases of babies who scream from start to finish and beyond. There are also cases when the baby is smiling and cheerful almost immediately after being freed.

Medically, the evidence for and against is almost perfectly balanced. The uncircumcised male has to be taught how to pull back the foreskin for proper cleansing. The lack can lead to infections. Yet parents of uncircumcised boys say that this is no problem. There are also risks of infection from the operation (slight).

By the best existing knowledge, you're facing a fifty-fifty decision, with neither choice being wrong or right. At the same time, it's not a decision to be made quickly or without thought. You and Mom may need to talk about it before coming to a mutual decision.

As with the name, the time to talk, research, and decide is before the birthing.

The Hospital Bag

There are actually two hospital bags—one for the mother and one for you. (The one for you is treated in the next section.) Both are similar in many ways, and both are determined by the circumstances, particularly your own bag. In both cases, the time to prepare is weeks, even months, before the predicted birth date. This doesn't mean that the bags actually have to be packed, just that all the things that will go in are ready so that you can pack and leave for the hospital in a matter of minutes. The onset of labor is not a great time to be starting the washing machine.

For the moment, think of the "hospital bag" as holding only those things that the mother needs. The basic rule of thumb is to keep it simple. This isn't a two-week camping trip. It's more likely to be two days or less, with many of the "conveniences of home" available (shower, soap, towels, etc.).

Should the required hospital stay become longer (e.g., there is the need for a C-section), she could be wearing hospital gowns through much of her stay and will still need only one change of street clothes. Besides, there will almost certainly be a chance for you to go home (after the birth) and get whatever was forgotten.

1. **Clothes:** She'll have the clothes she's wearing when you go to the hospital, but should have a complete change, including underwear, and perhaps even a second pair of shoes. Mom may also appreciate having a nursing bra (or two, for a change) at the hospital.

2. **Bedclothes:** Hospital gowns are famous for being uncomfortable and embarrassing. She'll probably wear one of these during the delivery, which is a good idea because giving birth tends to be messy and requires access. For recovery, a nice nightgown and robe can make the stay more pleasant. If the hospital won't allow the nightgown, a robe will serve as a cover-up. Keep in mind that she might be breast-feeding the new baby, and will probably require examinations. The front should open easily. Another part of "bedclothes" is a pair of slippers.

3. **Toiletries:** Most often the hospital will have soap, shampoo, and even toothpaste available (usually without additional charge). That doesn't mean your wife will want to use them. It's not unusual for her to have preferred brands. Many of these are available in travel-size containers. If not, small plastic containers are easy to find and are inexpensive. You can also find plastic containers for soap bars. Other toiletries include a brush or comb, makeup, toothbrush, perhaps a hair dryer . . . basically whatever she uses at home, but again keep in mind that the usual stay is no more than two days.

4. **Candies:** Labor can sometimes be long and hard. Some candy during it can give Mom some much-needed energy, and can also freshen her breath. It's a good idea to

check with the doctor first. Avoid anything and everything even mildly heavy. Snickers might be delicious, but
the nuts in it take some digestion. The muscles all through
her middle are going to be working very hard. There is a
risk of vomiting. This is why the mother is never fed even
during a long labor, and why her thirst is usually satisfied
with ice chips rather than cups of water.

5. **Mouthwash:** There is a very good chance that Mom's
   breath is going to get bad during the labor. If she vomits
   (which is not unusual), it can not only get worse, she can
   be uncomfortable from the taste in her mouth. A small
   bottle of mouthwash, and a container to spit it into, can
   be a relief and a refreshener.

6. **Lip Balm:** Many times an IV will provide fluids so Mom
   doesn't become dehydrated. Chances are good that the
   only liquid she'll be allowed will be ice chips. As the labor
   progresses, her lips may become chapped or feel dry. Lip
   balm can help relieve this.

7. **Miscellaneous:** This list could be almost endless. You
   might have been taught to use some kind of focal point,
   like a special picture or music (and the cassette player to
   play it, with fresh batteries). Maybe she likes to read, or
   have you read to her. It might be that you've been shown
   some massage techniques that use gloves, rollers, or other
   equipment. (It's also entirely possible that all your fine
   intentions and practice will never be used. A woman who
   has relished a massage during the pregnancy may
   scream at you during labor to not touch her.) Another
   important inclusion is a personal telephone book, with
   the names and phone numbers of those you want to inform immediately, from the hospital. Don't trust your
   memory.

The Daddy Bag

Your own bag should generally be kept separate. What goes in it depends on your circumstances. If your intention is to spend the entire time there in the hospital or other facility, you'll need a change of clothes, just as Mom will. You may need two changes. You will also need various toiletries for yourself. Some snacks will help you through the long labor. In short, if you intend to stay at the hospital, your own bag should be very much the same as hers.

It's not unusual for the mother to fall asleep during the labor. You could easily find yourself essentially alone and waiting for hours. During the recovery period she's likely to sleep more, or to be otherwise distracted. You'll be tired, too, but there may be times when you will want something to read.

Don't forget to pack some treats for yourself. Mom is the one doing the majority of the work, but that doesn't mean you're relaxing in a hammock in the shade. This doesn't mean that you should pack a picnic basket. Just don't forget that you might need an energy boost, especially during the labor when you don't want to leave the room.

You will probably also want a camera, still and/or video, with fresh film/tape and, where appropriate, flash, batteries, tripod, etc. Even if you have no desire to film the birth itself, you'll want to capture the moments afterward. (The nurse is almost certain to be accustomed to being asked to snap a picture or two.)

Getting Ready at Home

Your new child is going to be with you a long, long time. For a while the baby isn't going to be very interested in the new swing set or that shiny bicycle out in the garage. There are, however, some things that *will* be appreciated, and not just by the baby.

It's a common dream among new parents that baby is going to live in their bedroom with them. That's a nice idea—perhaps an excellent one for the first few weeks or even months—but it also gets old real fast for most people. It's not that love diminishes, nor does the desire to be with the baby. The reality is that both of you need some sleep.

In your room or elsewhere, your baby should have his or her bed. (It's not safe having the baby sleep in the same bed with you.) This bed should be located where the baby can nap without being disturbed, yet where you'll hear the cries. You'll find that babies sleep a lot! For a while, about all they seem to do is sleep, eat . . . and fill diapers. They need that sleep.

The bed must be safe. Babies and young children tend to move and roll in their sleep. They move around even more when awake. You need to be sure that your child won't fall out of bed, and also that there are no spots where fingers or toes can be pinched or injured. And you have to be sure that when the baby wakes, he won't be able to get out.

Some cribs are constructed so poorly that even a mildly active child will cause it to come apart. Others have sharp edges. A few (very rare these days) have paint that is dangerous. (Babies have the tendency to chew on just about anything.)

The inside of the crib is also important. Plastic sheets protect the mattress from stains, but also bring the danger of smothering. This is true even of those protective coverings that wrap all the way beneath the mattress. These can come loose. More commonly, they can tear, leaving dangerous openings.

This doesn't mean that you shouldn't use a protective cover. You'll not only protect the mattress, you'll be protecting the child. Urine, fecal matter, vomit, etc., can soak into the mattress. You won't be able to clean it away completely. That means stains, but it also means bacteria. Cleaning and sterilizing a protective mattress cover is far easier.

The key is to be sure that you have a good one that holds itself in place securely. Also be sure to inspect the cover on a regular basis. Look for tears or other damage. Replace the cover if need be.

If the baby is to sleep in a different room, consider using one of the monitoring devices available. These are basically just an intercom. Some have their own wires, others use the house wiring, and a few are wireless (they have a transmitter in the baby's room and a receiver wherever you happen to be).

You will also need a wide variety of other supplies. Diapers, either cloth (preferably with a service) or disposable, will be a constant need for the first couple of years. These come in a number of sizes. There is no need to plan ahead and stock diapers for six months in the future, but you should have at least one box of "newborn" diapers on hand *before* you go to the hospital.

You should also have at least three complete changes of clothing for the baby—more if you object to doing the laundry more than twice per day. (Even the best diapers leak.)

Don't worry about medicines for the baby. Rather, ask your doctor. This is not the time for self-diagnosis. Especially during that first year, even the common medications such as aspirin when used by someone without proper training can be dangerous. This also includes vitamins.

You should have a basic first aid kit. A baby thermometer is critical. This can be digital or of a more standard design (although glass is often not recommended). Either way, be sure to check the thermometer for accuracy on yourself. An inaccurate thermometer is more than useless. It's dangerous!

As a side note, the usual way to take a baby's temperature at home is beneath the arm. This takes a little more time, and you have to remember to add a degree to the reading.

(If the thermometer reads 98.6, the actual body temperature is 99.6.) But using the armpit is far safer than taking a reading in the mouth or anally.

For bathing you have a variety of choices. Keep safety in mind and you'll do fine. Remember that a wet, soapy, and squirmy baby can be quite slippery. Whatever method you use to keep your child clean, it has to bring with it maximum control.

A common solution is a baby's tub that fits into a sink. These are small (making it easier to keep control) and inexpensive. An advantage is that running water is right there at the sink, which minimizes cleanup afterward.

Soap and shampoo used should be pure. No deodorants, perfumes, or other additives. These are easy to find in just about any grocery or drugstore.

The foods you stock depend in part on how Mom intends to feed. If she's going to breast-feed, it might seem that you have everything and won't need bottles, nipples, and related supplies. Don't count on it.

It's a good idea to have *some* baby formula on hand. You will also need the sterile bottles, nipples, and caps, plus distilled water if the formula is the dry type. Even if Mom is breast-feeding, there could come times when she can't. Maybe she's ill. It's also possible that she'll develop some other condition that will prevent feeding this way. Or she might have to go somewhere, leaving you in charge. And don't forget those middle-of-the-night feedings. Sharing them not only gives Mom a much-needed rest, it gives you a very special sharing with your child.

A breast pump can be used to extract her own milk. The milk can be refrigerated, then warmed when it comes time to use it. Storage time is limited, however. A general rule is to use it the same day and no later than the next. It will probably last several days without problem, but there's no reason to risk your baby's health.

Whether you use formula or expressed breast milk, it's highly important that the containers are sterilized. Mere washing isn't enough. You can buy commercial sterilizers, but boiling works as well, and at less cost. Be sure to boil everything for at least five minutes.

A common mistake is the idea that babies love cow's milk. The truth is that many infants, and more than a few adults, can't handle it. Cow's milk is entirely different from human milk. It doesn't provide all the proper nutrients the baby needs and can be difficult to digest.

As time goes on, you'll find the need for a large variety of other things. The child needs toys, pacifiers, more clothes, and lots of miscellaneous things. Try to anticipate as best you can without going too far. Your major concern in preparing is to have the home prepared and ready for your new baby. All you really have to worry about right now involves what is needed in the first week or two.

If there are already children in the home, you may have some of the things you need. A crib used by your first child might be available for the newest addition. Bottles, especially those made of glass, can last for years. Nipples and caps wear out quickly, especially from being boiled to sterilize, but are inexpensive to replace. You might even have some unopened packages.

Take careful stock of what you have on hand. Some can be used. Some cannot.

Many new parents forget the car seat. It's dangerous to hold the baby while driving, and in most places it's also illegal. If there is an accident, the baby could go flying into the dash or through the windshield. To prevent this, the baby should be strapped securely into the car seat.

The best place for the car seat is in the middle of the backseat, with the back of the car seat facing forward. Don't just set it there. Strap it in tightly.

Childproofing

There's very little need to childproof right after the baby is born. It will be a while before the baby begins to crawl, and even longer before walking. Even so, this is the time to start thinking about it. Sooner than you realize, your newborn will be crawling around and getting into all sorts of trouble.

A classic technique is to get down on your hands and knees and crawl all around the house. That puts you closer to the child's level. Anything there that could even possibly present a risk needs attention. Some are obvious, some not. Always keep in mind that babies and young children are almost insatiably curious. They want to touch, and taste, just about anything they see.

All cleaners, chemicals, medicines, sharp objects, etc., have to be moved up out of reach. Don't trust "childproof" containers. Even babies can be ingenious at getting them open. It's easier and safer to move anything even remotely hazardous out of sight and out of reach.

Don't forget to check all rooms in the house. The kitchen alone isn't enough. Bathroom and laundry room cabinets very often contain potentially dangerous items.

Cabinet locks are readily available, cheap, and easy to install. For a while it may be inconvenient, but the protection is worth it. Even a baby of just a few months old and still crawling can get into lower cabinets.

One of the most common types is a spring-loaded plastic hook. The cabinet door closes, the hook snaps behind the cabinet edge. To open the cabinet, the door is opened partially and a spot on the hook is pushed to release it.

Another type is merely a flexible plastic hook. It works in exactly the same way. Although usually not quite as sturdy as the spring-loaded type, it works well.

In both cases, installation is easy. You merely align the hook on the cabinet door and attach it with screws.

There may be rooms in the house where you don't want a toddler to go. This will certainly include entry doors. (You don't want your young child wandering outside.) You could install actual locks on every door, but that's expensive, troublesome . . . and unnecessary.

A simple and inexpensive solution is to use doorknob protectors. These are usually made of plastic. They snap onto the doorknob. After that, a child's hand will merely spin the device. It takes a bit of pressure to squeeze enough to get a grip so the doorknob will turn. An adult will have little trouble. A young child will be unable to do it, except by sheer luck.

Some of these come with rubber inserts, kind of like a small button. The idea is that pushing down on this button puts the rubber into contact with the doorknob to make it easier to turn. While this is a good idea, it increases the chances that the child will be able to open that door. Consider removing those inserts.

Be aware that these same protectors can prevent others from using the doors. This can be of concern, for example, if you have an elder in the home, especially one who is suffering from arthritis in the hands.

What's for Dinner?

If you have the idea that you'll come home from the hospital with your new baby, and life will return to normal, forget it. Those first days in particular are going to be hectic. Mom needs her time to recover, to relax, and to spend time with the baby. So do you! Neither of you should be worrying about other things.

You can avoid a lot of the strain if you've followed the preceding advice about having the baby's room and/or crib ready, and have the basic supplies on hand. It will also help tremendously if you keep the house clean, at least during that last month. Your goal in general is to have as little to do as possible once you and the baby get home.

A part of that has to do with meals. Especially if she is breast-feeding, Mom needs good nutrition. So do you. Although fast and easy, the typical microwave dinner from the freezer section in the grocery store isn't usually known for being high in nutritional value.

You can have the same convenience by thinking, and preparing, ahead. Meals can be prepared and then frozen. Properly wrapped, these can even be prepared a month or more before the birth. Then, during those first days home, all you have to do is remove the meals from the freezer and pop them into the microwave or oven.

You can prepare any number of meals this way. Some keep better than others. Proper wrapping can be critical in all cases. Freezer burn can ruin otherwise excellent food, and can even make it dangerous to eat. This is less of a threat if the meal is stored for only a few weeks but is well worth consideration.

There are plenty of books available on canning and freezing that can help, but you don't really have to go to that extreme unless you want to. Your goal is simply to have two or three meals all set and ready to go. You may not appreciate the importance of this now, but with the new baby home, and your wife recovering, being able to spend just a minute or two to put dinner in to heat, as opposed to an hour just getting ready, is going to make a big difference.

A Clean House

It has been called "the nesting instinct." A fair number of (but not all) pregnant women exhibit it as the time for giving birth approaches. She suddenly seems to become overly concerned that everything is clean and everything is in place. Often she doesn't seem able to control it.

It tends to kick in a day or two before she goes into labor. This isn't a reliable indicator, however. Not all women experience this, nor can the timing be predicted. Some women become "clean freaks" the moment they learn that they are pregnant. Others may drive the father crazy by starting to clean the house just as he is trying to get her into the car and to the hospital.

Especially for a first-time mom, it is normal to want everything to be just right. Reason and rationality have little effect. What will help, however, is to put in a little extra effort on your own to keep the house clean throughout the pregnancy.

This is a nice thing to do regardless. As "the time" approaches, housework for her will become more and more difficult. It is usually recommended that she avoid anything heavy or strenuous in the last month and for several weeks after the birth. A major part of your job is to help her. Even if you've been doing your share of the housework all along, this is a time to do more than your share.

By making it routine, when the time comes to leave for the hospital, not much will be left to be done. The house will already be clean. Just as important, when the baby comes home, the house will be clean, and with the routine in place, it will stay clean.

Other Preparations

Many people have a separate "baby's room" and try to make it special for the new child in their home. The walls get a new coat of paint. Maybe the floor covering is replaced. In comes the new crib, with the new blankets, all the new toys, and new stuffed animals. What can also come is trouble.

The first trick is to make sure to safety-check everything.

Some toys aren't safe. Buttons come off and can be swallowed. There might be breakable parts, sharp edges, or other dangers. One child was rushed to the emergency room because he was choking. At the hospital a tiny sticker from the bottom of a toy was found in the child's throat.

Every toy, every piece of clothing, every decoration, every *everything*, needs to be checked carefully.

Repainting, reflooring, and more should be done far enough ahead of time so that all the fumes have completely disappeared well before the baby arrives.

One of the problems many first-time parents experience is preparing in the wrong ways. A common way is to have certain things ready, but for a child who is much older, not a newborn.

Actually, the needs of a newborn are fairly simple. Assuming that the child is in good health, much of the preparation is to make the situation easier on you and Mom. For example, the newborn won't really care that you have four or five dinners ready to go in the freezer, that all your laundry is done and hung up in the closet. The newborn isn't going to be impressed by the new linoleum you put down in the room, and even less impressed to know that it has a special coating that makes cleaning easier.

You can't possibly anticipate any of the special problems that might occur. Most of these are dictated by specific health problems. If you try to anticipate each and every possible variation, you'll only find yourself spending more than you need to on things that will never be used. It's just as easy to let yourself get carried away as it is to ignore the basic needs.

Planning for those first days or even weeks isn't difficult. Think of the necessities. Food. Clothing (including diapers). A place to sleep. Blankets. Cover those bases as best you can so that you can get by for at least a little while with minimal effort. This way you will have more time, and energy, to enjoy your new baby.

5

Old Wives' Tales (and Other Advice)

Joann was pregnant. Her mother, Betty, was thrilled. She'd been waiting to be a grandmother for some years. Now came her chance.

It was a grand time for both of them. They shared, both as mother and daughter, and as mother to mother. Betty, of course, was the expert in the latter. This was Joann's first. Betty had given birth to, and had raised, three children. And most of Betty's advice was sound.

One day Betty went along with her daughter to the doctor. Afterward they were to have a pleasant lunch together and then go shopping for some baby clothes.

The moment they stepped into the doctor's office, Betty let out a shriek, ripped off her coat, and pushed Joann back out the door, saying, "Don't look! Don't look!" Betty then rushed into the waiting room and threw her coat over the aquarium. She went back to Joann, took her lovingly by the hand, and said in a whisper, "He can't be much of a doctor to have a thing like that in here."

Joann was totally puzzled. "Mother, he's a very good doctor."

Betty shook her head. "If he were, he'd know." She pointed to the covered aquarium.

"What's wrong with having an aquarium, Mother? I have one at home. You seem to like it. You even helped me set it up."

"Yes, but yours has pretty fish. Thank goodness you don't have . . . one of those."

"One of what?" Joann asked.

"Then thank goodness you didn't see it. There was a big fish on the bottom. It was so ugly. Didn't your doctor tell you that if you look at something ugly, your baby will be born looking like it? You don't want your baby looking like an ugly fish, do you?"

Betty was an intelligent, well-educated woman. As with many of us (if not most), she merely held a belief without fact, and hadn't ever questioned it. Sometimes the cause of these beliefs is a lack of knowledge. Other times it's something that has been repeated so many times, it merely gets accepted without challenge.

It's possible that as the pregnancy progresses, you'll hear a number of old wives' tales. Some may even seem to make sense (and just might have some basis in fact). For example, there are several tales about cats.

When John's wife became pregnant for the first time, a well-meaning neighbor stopped by and told her in no uncertain terms that they had to get rid of all of their cats. "If you have a cat in the house with a new baby, it will get in the crib and suck out the baby's breath."

This isn't true, but there is some basis to it.

Cats sometimes seem to enjoy jumping into the crib with the baby, and will even snuggle around the baby's face. The smell of breast milk or formula can attract them. So can the warmth. A cat is unlikely to sleep in a bed with an adult human who moves and thrashes. But the baby is smaller, and tends to not move as much while sleeping. There is the possibility, however slight, that the cat can inadvertently smother the baby.

Couple this with the possibility of *SIDS—sudden infant death syndrome*. This condition is fortunately quite rare, but it does happen. The parent will put the baby to sleep. When returning a few hours later, the baby is dead for no apparent reason. Even the best physicians and scientists aren't completely sure what causes this. One theory is that the baby basically "forgets" to breathe.

If a cat has been in the crib, there is going to be the temptation (and a valid one) to blame it on the cat.

Another potential danger is toxoplasmosis. This disease is caused by a microscopic protozoan called *Toxoplasma gondii*. A mild case may not be noticed. A more severe infection can be extremely troublesome or even fatal, especially in an infant. If Mom contracts the disease while pregnant, there can be even greater complications.

This protozoan is found in mammals and birds, but the feces of a cat are the most common source. (The same is true of the bottom of a birdcage.) It also comes from undercooked meat, especially pork but also beef and lamb.

There is no reason to get rid of the pets, however. The mother should simply avoid any contact with the litter box or with soil outside the cat may have used. Obviously, keep the newborn away from these as well. The same is true of other pets. Cleanliness is critical. If a litter box is used, be sure to keep it clean. (It's best if you do this. There is only a distant chance of catching the disease, and in that rare instance, treating it in you is far easier, with far fewer risks, than treating it in an infant, or in a pregnant or nursing mother.)

Also, if you like rare meat, at least for now change your

tastes and be sure it is thoroughly cooked. (Because of the danger, consider changing on a more permanent basis.)

Cats also scratch and bite. Both can cause infections. Other pets can bring on similar dangers. Caution is necessary and prudent. (And don't forget that young children are often a danger to the pet.)

Another common belief that may have basis in fact is the value of exposing the baby to music, reading, and talking, both while it is in the womb and after. Many claim that these things can make the baby more calm and more intelligent.

Studies so far are inconclusive. However, it is known that the unborn is able to react to sound as early as the fourth month and definitely by the sixth. There are strong indications that the newborn reacts differently to the voices of the mother and father, which signifies a learned familiarity. There is also some evidence that the tone of the conversations can make a difference. Although it's uncertain, it's possible that the unborn might react to the calm words of a loving couple much differently than to the loud arguments of a couple not getting along.

After the birth, the child learns the language by repetition. The baby hears words over and over again and will eventually be able to mimic them. It doesn't matter which language it is—English, Spanish, Chinese, Russian—the baby will absorb the language with amazing ease. Imagine a child that is raised in total silence. It has nothing to mimic. Compare this to a child that hears nothing but baby talk, consisting of higher-pitched and often mispronounced words and phrases. Then compare that to a child who has both parents speaking normally, and often.

Even as the child grows and learns, if he hears only baby talk, his learning can be held back. (Much the same can happen if the language used is always so far above the child's ability that little or nothing can be learned.)

The effect of music is less certain yet. Even with adults, one person is calmed and soothed by a Mozart concerto, while another is bored or even irritated. The same can be said of any style or type of music.

The general rule of thumb established by studies says what is fairly obvious. Slower, calmer, quieter music tends to be more soothing. Faster, more energetic, and louder music tends to be energizing. Simpler tunes, like simpler words, tend to be more easily absorbed. Make of this what you wish. You'll find experts on every side ready to agree or to disagree.

The only truly known fact is that overly loud music can cause damage to the eardrums. The baby in the womb gets a natural muffling from Mom's body, but the unborn can still suffer potential damage. For the newborn, overly loud sounds can cause a lifetime of damage.

One final widely accepted myth that is based on fact is that the pregnant woman is delicate and needs to be "treated with kid gloves."

Throughout this book you'll be encouraged to provide all the love, understanding, and support you can. This is important. It doesn't mean you should bend to every whim. It certainly doesn't mean that you should become a slave. That's not good for you or for her.

Recognize that her body is going through a variety of changes. She can't always help how she acts or feels, any more than you could if your body were being put through the same kinds of changes. Many of these changes are more physical in nature. Especially if she has had, and continues to have, a poor diet, the growing fetus draws on her body for growth. Even the most healthy of women are still providing life support for two bodies. This doesn't mean that she is helpless.

During the first trimester, the "kid gloves" applies mostly to supplying much-needed psychological support and understanding. The "delicateness" comes mostly from her hormones causing major changes in her body.

Unless there is a problem, through both the first and second trimesters, Mom is physically capable of doing just about anything she could normally. In fact, coddling her too much can actually cause harm. If you do everything for her—treat her as being too helpless—she might take on that attitude. Worse, she might lack some valuable and necessary physical exercise just when she needs it most.

Later in the pregnancy, even some simple tasks are going to become more difficult. Her weight is up, her balance is off; bending over to put on shoes means trying to get around a massive bulge in her middle. It's not unusual for her to feel uncomfortable all the time. It's also not unusual for her to feel somewhat helpless. Things she could normally do, she can't without effort—or can't do at all.

On another level, there are certain things Mom should avoid. Heavy lifting is perhaps the most common example. Because of her changed balance, this is more difficult to begin with. It can also cause the abdominal muscles to separate. Hernias and hemorrhoids are also more common.

Yes, Mom is more delicate, particularly late in the pregnancy. But unless there are complications, she's not helpless. Mostly it's a matter of being aware and of using common sense. One extreme is to pretend that nothing is different, with Mom working as hard as ever. The other extreme is turning Mom into a bed-ridden patient. (Note that the latter might be necessary in some cases. Follow the doctor's advice.)

Gender and Twins

There are a number of theories for determining the gender and the number of babies being carried. Some of these reach back into conception itself. Many are contradictory. One claims that if you want a boy child, the woman should lie on her left side during intercourse. Another claims just as strongly that the way to do it is to have her lie on her right side. Another says that to have a boy the couple should be east to west in bed, and north to south for a girl. Still another says she should be on the bottom, while yet another says she should be on the top. One version even advises that Mom should stand on her head after intercourse if she wants a boy.

If you want twins, have intercourse under a full moon. But having intercourse under a full moon can cause your children to be unruly, or according to another theory, makes them more susceptible to the influence of Satan. A softer version says that this will cause the children to look like animals.

There are literally hundreds of these stories and myths, and variations of each.

One tells of how to determine the gender of the child by holding a needle on a thread over Mom's stomach. If the needles swings back and forth in a straight line, she'll have a boy. If the needle moves in a circle, it will be a girl. A variation of this gives the same directions but claims that a wedding ring is needed, not a needle. One more rare version calls for a kernel of corn.

If the tummy bulge sticks out more, it's a boy (because boys lie in the front of the stomach, according to this tale). A girl has the weight more evenly spread, and so doesn't bulge as much.

One woman told me, "Morning sickness is worse when the mother is carrying a female child. Carrying a boy makes for an easy, joyful pregnancy." In an interview the very next day, another woman told me exactly the opposite.

"If the woman gets large quickly, she'll have twins."

"A woman who is fat will have twins."

"If you have sex twice in the same night that conception takes place, you will have twins."

Depending on your definition of "large," the first is possibly true, depending on other conditions. As should be obvious, a woman carrying multiple babies is likely to be larger. This doesn't mean overweight, but large in the uterus. If Mom does become large in this regard, quickly or otherwise, the doctor is very likely to monitor it. It could mean that there is more than one baby growing inside. It could also indicate some other problem—or none at all. Regardless, the doctor will want to know, which is why fetal growth is watched so carefully.

Being overweight, however, has nothing to do with it. A genetic predisposition within the family to having twins might come with another predisposition to being overweight, but to the best of existing scientific knowledge, a woman who is overweight going into a pregnancy is likely to have certain problems. Twins is not necessarily one of them.

The third tale has nothing at all to do with it. As stated in Chapter One, the sperm make their way through the cervix, then divide into two groups. By this time, most of the sperm have already died. Of the half (approximately) that accidentally end up in the correct side, only a few make it to the egg. The moment a sperm penetrates the outer coat, the egg is sealed off. No other sperm will be able to penetrate. Conception has already taken place.

The total journey from vagina to egg takes a while. Although it's possible for sperm to survive for as long as forty-eight hours, even this becomes irrelevant. Assume that the egg is there and ready to be fertilized. Assume intercourse and the introduction of sperm. Assume a second intercourse in the same evening (or afternoon, or whenever). It doesn't matter. The first sperm that reaches the egg and penetrates completes conception, and the egg is sealed. Any additional sperm that manage to make it that far will be beating on the proverbial brick wall and locked door.

Some Less Likely Stories

Michael was a science teacher. An eclipse was about to occur. He'd set up a telescope with camera equipment attached to photograph the event. His wife, Diane, was always interested in what her husband was doing. Since they'd been married seven years, she'd learned more about science than in all her years in school, and found it fascinating.

Her mother was horrified when she heard about this. She held the belief that looking at an eclipse, solar or lunar, would cause the child to be born with a cleft palate.

Similar to the "fish story" at the beginning of this chapter is the tale of how you shouldn't hold anger against someone because if you do, your child will be born looking like that person. Not far from that is the warning that pregnant women should ignore their food cravings. Why? Because if they give in, the child will be born with a birthmark in the shape of the food the woman craved.

It's possible that this came about because the typical birthmark doesn't have a distinctive shape. This becomes like seeing shapes in the stars. Most can see a fairly definite pan shape in the Big Dipper. Look at Orion and you can see the hourglass shape that could be taken as a person who is per- haps wearing a togalike garment with a belt, and even with the scabbard of a sword. You may not recognize all the parts, but it doesn't take much to see Scorpio as the stars' image of a scorpion.

Other constellations are less distinct and require more imagination. This hasn't stopped people from drawing the pictures, or making the stories.

A birthmark might truly have a yellow tint, and could even look like a banana if you squint just right. Other people might even see it the same way, if you tell them what it's supposed to be. They could just as easily think it's a fish, a crescent moon, or even a shapeless blob (which it often is).

Again, it doesn't matter. Craving bananas might actu- ally reflect nothing more than her body recognizing a need for potassium, or just for a favorite sweet. No matter what, that craving in itself is not going to result in a birthmark of any shape.

A father I interviewed was very serious when he told me that if you tickle baby before it can laugh, the child will grow up to stutter or be totally mute. He offered as proof a lifelong friend of his who stuttered, and who was still struggling with the problem. He pointed out that his friend's parents were always very loving and playful. His "logical deduction" was that they must have always been this way, therefore must have tickled the baby, and since the baby grew into a boy who stuttered, this particular myth was "proven" to be true.

He'd left out a number of points.

First, no one really knows for certain why a person stutters. There can be many causes, not the least of which is a growing child who is made to feel insecure. A child with loving, playful parents is *less* likely to feel this.

Second, most babies seem to enjoy being tickled (at least at times) and love to laugh. Often it's the tickling that teaches them how. No matter how funny the joke, a two-month-old infant is highly unlikely to laugh at the punch line. They will, however, learn laughter and pleasure during play and tickling.

Third, if this myth were true, either very few parents play with and tickle their babies, or there are millions of people who can somehow hide stuttering very well.

Stories of good luck and bad luck are also common—especially those concerning bad luck. This is probably because when everything goes smoothly, no one really notices—but when things go badly, people begin looking for a cause. In the distant past, many accepted the notion that when something bad happened, it was because the individual(s) did something to offend the gods.

It has been said that if you select the baby's name before the birth, you're inviting disaster. The same applies to bringing any baby supplies into the home beforehand. There is a connection with reality, but this goes back to not noticing the good, and looking for the causes of the bad.

Millions of parents give birth to children every year. Although there are no statistics, it's a good chance that many of these discuss the baby's name and start preparing the home. In all of this, there will be times when the pregnancy goes wrong. The parents will have a name that serves only to be carved into a tombstone, or a bedroom filled with a crib, diapers, and other supplies for a baby that will never come.

This is heartbreaking, of course. Coming home from the hospital with such terrible news and facing a room you've worked so hard to prepare can make the loss that much worse.

However, this doesn't prove the correlation between thinking or planning ahead and disaster. Yes, it can happen. Even with the best conditions, circumstances, and medical expertise, what seems to be a perfect pregnancy can go wrong. If it does, the cause is almost certainly some problem that wasn't diagnosed, or that couldn't be. It's not because you picked a name or bought some diapers.

Honest Questions?

As the two of you go through this, you're likely to be handed a lot of advice. Don't turn your back on it lightly. Even when it doesn't make sense, accept that the person offering it just might know something—or if not, that these tales sometimes have at least *some* basis in fact. Also recognize three other factors.

One is that some people (most, if you tend toward pessimism) have the tendency to exaggerate, dramatize, and expand. (Pass it through the rumor mill and the new fifty-five-year-old lady delivering mail in the neighborhood can end up being a redheaded seductress barely out of high school seen sneaking around Mr. Simon's door.)

Another is that people like to feel important and knowledgeable. This can sometimes bring about the exaggeration and expansion.

The third, and perhaps most important, factor is that the

vast majority of the people who offer advice—or who ask silly questions—actually do mean well. It's not always easy accepting this.

Bill and his wife, Sara (eight months pregnant), were out at a movie. In the lobby two women walked over with large smiles. "Are you pregnant?" one asked, while reaching out to put her hands on Sara's stomach.

The other also ran her hands over Sara's stomach. "It's a boy," she announced. "You can tell because of how high it is right here." With that she tapped firmly on the top of Sara's tummy. Then the woman turned to Bill, then back to Sara as though he weren't really there. "Is this the father?"

Both Sara and Bill were a bit dumbfounded, but it got worse. A third woman came over, dragging her husband behind. "Ohhhh," she squealed. "When is the child due?"

All this was followed by a series of questions.

"Was the child planned?"

"How long have you tried?"

"Are you *sure* this is the father?"

"What kind of job does he have?"

"Do you want a boy or a girl?"

"Have you considered the baby's college education?"

"How long have you been married? You *are* married, aren't you?"

Bill and Sara bowed out as quickly and as politely as they could when the third woman began pressing her husband forward to feel the baby move.

This story is true, but is hopefully an exaggeration of what you might face. Most of the time you'll get smiles and pleasant comments. Those who feel the urge to touch Mom's tummy will usually restrain themselves. There will be plenty of people who offer advice. Even when the advice or questions seem strange, impolite, or intrusive, keep in mind that the vast majority come from good intentions.

After the Birth

Be prepared for the advice and stories to continue after the baby is born. They might even come more often. Even people who have never had children are often full of advice and stories.

One couple was warned by a neighbor to do everything they could to keep their child from walking before she was twelve months or older. "A baby who walks earlier than that will be bowlegged for life," the neighbor claimed. "The child will probably need leg braces!"

Many children are born almost bald. Others have a full head of hair. The mother of a child who'd been born with hair proudly informed her best friend, who'd given birth to a bald baby, that she should lather and shave the baby's head regularly. "It stimulates hair growth. If you don't do it now, your boy will become bald later."

One of the more unusual interviews was with a woman who had an eight-year-old who was still breast-feeding. The child would eat a regular dinner, but would breast-feed almost as a dessert. He wasn't allowed to unless his behavior that day was perfect. At the opposite end of this spectrum are claims that breast-feeding beyond six months (or at all) causes a breast fixation that can lead to abuse.

Somewhat allied is the woman in her late fifties who firmly advised her thirty-five-year-old daughter that the newborn's inability to sleep through the night was due to an allergy to breast milk. She may have had the right idea, but the wrong source of milk. It's not unusual for a baby, or an adult, to have trouble with cow's milk. It can cause indigestion. Human breast milk, on the other hand, has been justifiably called the perfect food for human babies.

Even while your new baby is still in diapers, you're almost

bound to hear all sorts of advice, theories, methods, etc., on how to raise children. And how to discipline them. Some believe in being firm and strict. Others feel that the child should have nearly total freedom and no punishments at all.

Don't be too surprised if the strongest notions come from those who have never had children. The lack of real-life experience perhaps allows notions to develop, while that same lack doesn't provide the chance to see firsthand things that just don't work. This makes it easy to become set on an idea. (And sometimes those ideas aren't so bad! The perspective of distance can sometimes provide some valuable insight.)

What you're likely to find is that even your own best ideas will go through needed modifications. What works for a while may stop working. What works for one child may not work with another. Basically there are few hard-and-fast rules. Most of it is common sense, blended with a *lot* of patience. (You'll need some of that patience just to deal with all the well-meaning people who offer advice and stories.)

Every situation is different. So is every child. Your job as a parent is to sift through all the input, and be prepared to accept some, reject some, adapt some, change some. Beyond that, just do the best you can.

6

The First Few Months

$\mathcal{F}$or many, the first few months aren't dramatic. Some women don't even know they're pregnant for the first two to three months. This is especially true if she has a history of irregular or missed periods.

On the other hand, some women go through drastic changes even early in the pregnancy. A common symptom is morning sickness, which doesn't necessarily happen in the morning. She (and you) might find herself becoming more moody. There might be cravings for certain foods. It's fairly common for her breasts to become sensitive, even painful.

Mom is obviously going to be going through many changes during the pregnancy. In the first few months you may not be able to see them, but they're happening. Her body actually begins to go through some major changes from the moment of conception.

In general, her hormones go through shifts every month

from puberty to menopause. After fertilization of the egg, this cycle is replaced by another. These shifts cause changes in her body, in her hormones, and in her moods.

Weight Gain

All healthy pregnant women gain weight. She is supposed to. In fact, if she doesn't, the doctor is going to become very concerned very quickly. This gain is much more than just the weight of the child and supportive tissues. Most doctors will recommend that Mom gain somewhere between twenty-two and twenty-seven pounds, depending on the individual, with the average weight of the newborn being roughly eight pounds. Almost all of this will be put on in the last months at a rate of about one pound per week, but it often begins during the first trimester.

It's very common for the will-be-mother to feel "fat and dumpy" even before it begins to show. Toward the end of the pregnancy she possibly weighs more than she has ever weighed in her life, which makes the feeling more understandable. Before this, however, the changes her body is undergoing can cause the feeling. Often water retention makes the face and arms puffy, giving the appearance—or feeling— of being fat. All your reassurances won't seem to be a whole lot of help.

You can tell her on a daily basis how beautiful she is. You can point out the studies that show that statistically the male finds a pregnant woman to be very attractive. You can even mention all the extra attention she gets from everyone, including total strangers (and including some innocent flirtation by the men around her). And *still* she'll go on and on about how fat and unattractive she is. "I'm not attractive," she might say, "I'm fat!"

"You're not fat. You're pregnant!" is a good answer, but even that may not work. Even so, don't stop telling her. Those reassurances may not seem to be doing any good, but they are. (Whatever you do, don't try anything like, "I don't care how fat you are, I still love you.")

Above all, keep in mind that pregnancy is *not* the time for Mom to go on a diet to lose weight (unless the doctor recommends it). Literally, she's eating for two. What she eats, or does not eat, affects the baby and the baby's healthy growth. (See "Importance of Diet" in this chapter.)

It's also not the time to go on eating binges. Pregnancy can (but doesn't always) bring on cravings. The doctor will be checking her weight at every visit, starting from the beginning. It's normal and necessary for her to put on three times the weight of the child or more during the pregnancy. The problem comes when the weight gain becomes excessive. This isn't good for her or for the child.

You might think it's nice, and a show of affection, to bring her candies, ice cream, and other sweets. It is. Too often, however, it can be harmful to both the mother and the child. Candy is high in calories, but not of much nutritional value.

This is the time to pay attention to a balanced diet. For both of you. Giving in to some occasional cravings is fine. Doing so constantly isn't good, and may be a sign that there is something lacking in the normal diet.

The doctor may suggest vitamin/mineral supplements. This might be multiple vitamin capsules, or could be something specific. Follow these instructions. Do *not* try to "prescribe" on your own. It's unlikely that taking vitamins will cause any problems, but the doctor should know, and approve.

The same applies to any medications, even aspirin. Find out early what the doctor will allow and what he won't. What does this have to do with diet? It's fairly common for a pregnant woman to feel nauseated, or to experience flatulence and/or constipation. Before you get out one of the common remedies, you should know which ones are approved by the doctor. More, find out if perhaps there isn't a natural way to control these problems—namely a change in the diet. The doctor is unlikely to be a dietitian or nutritionist, but he will probably have some suggestions.

Water Retention

A fair amount of the weight gain is water retention. It is caused by several factors especially increased levels of the hormones progesterone and estrogen. This is also one of the reasons her breasts may become sensitive.

In most cases this isn't a serious problem, but it can be, especially in the later months. One effect is that she might get a bloated, puffy feeling, which often increases her notion that she's fat. Another is a condition called edema, which shows up as swelling, especially in the legs but elsewhere, too.

The chances of her suffering from edema early in the pregnancy are slight, but this is when you need to begin awareness of it. It's easier to treat if caught early. Treatment, of course, is a matter for the doctor.

There is one thing you can do, and early. This is to reduce the amount of salt in your diet (which means her diet as well). If you're used to salting everything, break the habit. Too much salt isn't good for you in any case. It also aggravates the problem of water retention. By using less salt in the diet, you're helping both general health and water retention.

Many of the convenient foods are already high in salt content. Soups, canned vegetables, frozen dinners, fast foods, and many more have what most doctors consider to be an excess of salt. Look for products that are "low salt" or "low sodium."

Even if water retention seems to be a problem, do NOT reduce the amount of fluid intake. Not unless the doctor orders, which is highly unlikely. Fluids are important. This means clean water, fruit juices, etc., not beer, wine, or even coffee.

Mood Swings

Mom is going through a lot right now, in addition to hormonal influences. She may have desperately wanted to have a baby. The two of you may have been trying for some time. The reality of *being* pregnant, however, can be frightening. You may feel some of this yourself. The baby is coming. The two of you are going to be parents, responsible for the new life and all that comes with it. You might worry about finances, or if the baby will be healthy.

These and other worries affect the woman at least as much, and usually more. She may suddenly wonder if you really even want the child, or if you regret having gotten her pregnant. Especially as she gains weight, she may even wonder if you still love her.

Mom is likely to have another fear. No matter how supportive and helpful you are, *she* is the one who is pregnant. It's her body that is caring for the life inside her. Every little twinge can make her afraid that she's going into a miscarriage. Her concerns about the general health of the fetus are almost certainly going to be stronger than your own. She lives with it, day by day, even minute by minute, inside her own body.

She could be worried about going through the pregnancy, especially the later months. She is likely to be worried about the birthing itself. Some describe this process as "discomfort." It's a lucky woman who faces so little. In most cases, giving birth hurts, plain and simple. She's the one who will be going through it.

Recognize your own similar fears. Whether you discuss them together depends on your relationship. Sometimes it helps if she knows that she's not alone in these fears, and that you have them yourself. It can even create a tighter bond between you. At the same time, it can be a delicate subject that requires a careful balance. A positive attitude for both of you is important. Be supportive.

She should feel free to talk to you about things that are bothering her. And you should be as understanding as you can, not judgmental. Sometimes she's looking for answers. More often she merely needs someone to talk to—a way to express what she's feeling. It's not easy to know when to attempt an answer, and when to listen mostly in silence.

One fairly common mood swing that can be truly puzzling is depression. "I should never have become pregnant." You, and she, can try your best to find the cause, without luck. There might even be a reason other than a shifting of the hormones in her body. Again, all you do is be supportive. If the depression seems very bad, or lasts more than a few days, talk to the doctor. This is one time you don't need her permission. She may not give it. But be absolutely sure that there is a valid reason for concern. (Could she be mad at you for some good cause?)

There is probably no reason for concern, but at least you've told the doctor so he is aware of the situation, and can verify that nothing is wrong.

Not all of the mood swings are negative, by the way. At times she might become almost giddy. Other times she might have a stronger sex drive than ever before. She could develop a sudden love of cleaning and cooking. It's even possible that she'll decide that this is a great time to go back to school or take up a new hobby.

The key, once again, is to be supportive. That doesn't mean to be "wimpy." This rarely helps, and can make matters worse. The time may come when the right action is to stand up for yourself. The dividing line between the two is never very clear, so make such decisions cautiously and intelligently.

Physical and emotional energy is decreased during pregnancy. Mom should avoid stress as much as possible. She should also have a time each and every day to relax, whether that be to take a nap, read a magazine, or whatever. Take a calm walk together and just talk. You'll become closer, get the chance to know each other even better, and it's good for Mom, both for the exercise and for the relaxation. (It's also good for Dad!)

Morning Sickness

Whatever the cause of morning sickness about 50 percent of all pregnant women suffer from it to one extent or another. (Other sources claim that as many as 70 percent get it.) It tends to be worse in women pregnant for the first time, and for those who are carrying more than one baby. Generally, it begins after about a month and subsides in the second trimester.

Normally it is no real problem. It's uncomfortable, to be sure, but it usually ends after a few weeks and presents no danger. The best thing you can do during this time is to offer as much understanding as possible. It will pass. (If it doesn't, the doctor should be notified.)

Mom isn't really sick, but she wakes up with a queasy stomach and feeling like she has the flu. It could be that certain odors set off an attack, especially tobacco, coffee, or fried foods. The taste of certain foods might also set it off. Keep in mind that she's not doing it on purpose. She can't help it.

Mild morning sickness is often helped by her snacking on some dry crackers (preferably low-salt) or unbuttered toast first thing in the morning before even standing up. Frequent and small meals during the day can also help.

If you're off to work all day, there won't be much you can do to help out then. However, you *can* make sure that there are crackers in the house. Maybe you can even bring them to her before you head off for work. If Mom also works, the extra effort on your part becomes even more important. One father took to slipping a Baggie of crackers into his wife's purse each morning, along with a short, romantic note. Also remember that a working mother needs extra help at home. If you handle more of the household chores, she will be less fatigued. That in itself helps reduce morning sickness.

There is some evidence that vitamin B_6 can help to a certain extent. (It also seems to be critical in the early stages of the baby's growth and even before conception to prevent congenital malformations.) Vitamin supplements, such as the prenatal multiple vitamins, can help. Natural food sources—a good diet—also helps. Nicely enough, B_6 is found most abundantly in the same foods that provide the needed protein and other goodies. Meats, cereal grains, and wheat germ are all excellent sources. (Note: Do *not* self-prescribe anything, including vitamins!)

You can also help by finding out what seems to trigger her nausea and avoid those things for a while. You might have a fondness for morning coffee, but the smell makes Mom feel ill. No big deal. Switch to tea for a couple of weeks, or get your morning coffee at work, or on the way. The condition won't last very long.

There seems to be strong evidence that a well-rounded and balanced diet *prior* to conception can greatly reduce, and possibly eliminate, morning sickness. If you're reading this during the planning stages of pregnancy (she's not yet pregnant), start now by making sure that your diets are sound. The healthier Mom is ahead of time, the better all of it will go, and the better the chances of having a healthy baby.

As the fetus grows, it's going to be taking in the nutrients it needs to grow, which depletes the mother's own supply. If the needed nutrients aren't there to begin with, and aren't supplied during the pregnancy, the baby won't be getting enough, and Mom is going to suffer as well.

Severe morning sickness, called *hyperemesis gravidarum*,

can become serious. If Mom is vomiting and not eating, she can suffer a drastic weight loss. This just at the time when her body needs to gain weight and to have a balanced diet.

A little vomiting is probably okay. If it's violent and/or daily, it would be a good idea for her to see the doctor. Meanwhile, be sure that Mom has plenty of fluids to help prevent dehydration and to reduce the acidity in the stomach. (That acidity will induce further vomiting and could cause gastric ulcers.)

Don't wait if it seems serious. See the doctor right away, or at least call.

Other Changes

A wide variety of changes can be expected. It's unlikely that all of the following will happen. Perhaps none of it will. Your goal is merely to be aware of what *could*. Most of the time the symptom will be minor, but awareness gives you the needed edge so that the doctor can be informed if the situation becomes worse.

Perhaps the most common symptom is fatigue. This is understandable. A new life is growing inside her body. To make this possible, her own body is changing. More blood is being made (up to about a 50 percent increase in volume), and about 15 percent more oxygen is needed. Heart rate increases by ten to fifteen beats per minute. Nutrition must satisfy her usual needs, plus what is needed for the pregnancy.

Fatigue is common in the first trimester, then usually fades through the second trimester, only to come back again as full term nears. Don't expect Mom to tell you about it. Pay close attention on your own. Take on a few more household chores. Do your best to see that she gets plenty of rest.

Dizziness, headaches, and even faintness are all fairly common in the early months. Don't become overly concerned, but do pay close attention. Chances are good that the causes are fatigue, hormonal changes, changes in the circulatory system, and also changes in dietary needs. However, these symptoms can also be a sign of another problem, such as *ectopic pregnancy*.

An ectopic pregnancy is when the fertilized egg attaches itself somewhere other than inside the uterus. Most often this happens in the fallopian tube, which is why this kind of pregnancy is sometimes called a tubal pregnancy. This is potentially life-threatening. The uterus is well suited for a growing baby. The fallopian tube, abdomen, or cervix is not. It doesn't take long before the growing baby causes the surrounding tissues to push outward and burst. This causes internal bleeding.

If the headaches and dizziness are accompanied with vaginal bleeding, she should see the doctor immediately. The same is true if they are severe or continue. There is only a seven in one thousand chance of the pregnancy being ectopic, and most of these occur in women over thirty-five or who have a history of ectopic pregnancies, surgery on a fallopian tube, several abortions, or who have had a pelvic infection. Of all ectopic pregnancies, only one in twenty-five hundred prove fatal, with the majority of those being because the parents-to-be ignored the symptoms or were dishonest with the doctor.

Also be aware that *slight* vaginal bleeding ("spotting") is fairly common. Roughly 20 percent of all pregnant women "spot" in the first trimester. If this occurs very early in the pregnancy, such as within a week to ten days of conception, it could be caused by the egg implanting itself in the uterus. There may be other causes as well. The initial examination will probably include a Pap smear. This very often causes spotting.

Slight spotting probably doesn't call for a rush to the emergency room. Heavier or continued bleeding, especially if accompanied by cramping or pain in the pelvic region probably does. In any case, even slight spotting should be mentioned to the doctor. The rule of thumb is that if it's slight and lasts less than a day, it's probably safe to wait until the next regular visit. If it lasts more than a day, call right away for advice. If it's heavy bleeding, or even moderate, don't wait. If this is accompanied by a fever, chills, or pain, get to the hospital NOW!

Eyesight may change during pregnancy. It will probably return to normal shortly after the birth, and could even straighten itself out during the pregnancy itself. This is usually not much of a problem, but if it seems that glasses are needed, the situation is severe enough to warrant letting the doctor know.

Increase in tooth decay and gum disease are both common, and fortunately are both easily solved. Hygiene and a good diet are the key. Related is *ptyalism*, or increased salivation. This condition sometimes increases nausea. Brushing the teeth often, rinsing the mouth, sucking on peppermints, all help. Cutting down on starchy foods and sugar can also help.

Hair growth may increase, and hair might become thicker. It might even start growing in places that are usually relatively bald. It will also tend to be oilier. At the other end, if Mom loses hair, or if hair seems to be getting drier and more brittle, check the diet.

Expect her skin to become oilier. She may even get pimples. Moles and dark spots might also develop. Some fear that the sudden appearance is a sign of cancer. Although it's always best to have the doctor check, keep in mind that it's all probably very normal.

She may also get stretch marks in her skin, particularly on the breasts and across the abdomen. Vitamin E and lanolin may help some, but a balanced diet is better. Chances are pretty good that the stretch marks will stay, at least during the pregnancy, no matter what you do.

The breasts are likely to change size and shape, especially

later in the pregnancy. Support for breasts, such as with a special bra, can help. Obviously you can't select this for her. All you can do is suggest. Correct fit is important. Also expect a degree of increased tenderness.

Water retention can cause her feet and ankles to swell. Don't be surprised if her shoes don't fit. The main caution here is to be aware of the swelling. Minor swelling is normal. You can probably take care of it with a good foot, ankle, and leg massage (which Mom will appreciate!). More extensive swelling could be a more severe and troublesome case of edema that needs the doctor's attention.

Backaches are very common in the later stages of pregnancy, and may occur in the early stages. Regardless, this is a good time to begin preparation to prevent them later on. Exercise is one solution. You can also take this opportunity to practice giving back rubs. (See the Appendix on "Massage.")

The vagina often begins to secrete more fluid. She shouldn't douche! Not without specific doctor's orders. This can kill off good bacteria and can in turn cause an infection. If the vagina has a bad odor that a simple shower doesn't wash away, talk to the doctor.

Expect her to have an increased need to urinate. Frequent urination is caused by relaxing bladder muscles, increase in level of progesterone, and pressure from the expanding uterus. This tends to decrease during middle pregnancy and return in the last months.

What should be obvious but so often isn't, for some reason, is the increase in fatigue. Her body is going through a lot. Inside her is a new life that is growing and taking nutrients. Despite the increase in her blood supply and respiration, being pregnant can be very tiring.

You can help. Your job is to absorb some of the daily chores and strains. Don't make a big deal of it. Certainly don't come off as though Mom is so delicate, tender, and helpless that she can't vacuum the floor or wash the dishes. Everyone enjoys pampering. No one enjoys being treated as helpless. Don't expect to be told over and over how wonderful *you* are for taking out the trash or making the bed. It is far more effective and meaningful to simply do those chores, without being asked and without need for praise.

The Importance of Diet

Diet has been mentioned a number of times in this chapter. As an old expression goes, "You are what you eat." There's more truth to this than you might realize. For example, if you have a diet that is high in fat and salt, you can expect heart, artery, and blood pressure problems later in life. Or to exaggerate, imagine having a diet that consists entirely of Snickers candy bars and vodka.

Protein is the basic building block. Animal products, such as meat and milk, are generally of the highest quality. Vegetable proteins are of lower quality and more difficult for the body to use. This doesn't mean that if you are vegetarian, you should suddenly change your ways. However, be aware that the need for protein goes up by about 50 percent during pregnancy. She will need, per day, approximately forty-six milligrams to seventy-six milligrams during pregnancy and sixty-six milligrams during lactation (breast-feeding).

Iron is always important in a woman's diet due to her menstrual cycle. It's easy for a woman to become anemic. During pregnancy the need for iron becomes even more important. Her body has to provide all the blood for her system (increased by as much as 50 percent during pregnancy), as well as the blood for the baby.

A fairly common problem during pregnancy is *anemia*, which is a low level of hemoglobin in the blood. (Hemoglobin is an iron-containing protein.) For the first few months of the baby's life, the entire iron supply is built-in having been stored during pregnancy. It's common for the doctor to prescribe iron supplements because it is difficult to get all the needed iron from diet alone.

Dry beans contain both protein and iron. Dark green vegetables, which also give vitamin A, also tend to be good sources of iron. Whole grains and enriched foods are other sources.

Women in particular are prone to osteoporosis, a painful and sometimes crippling bone disease in which the bones become brittle. Calcium builds bones and teeth and also helps in reducing hypertension (high blood pressure). Milk is the primary source in our standard diet. The need for milk doubles during pregnancy and nursing.

The average adult needs about 800 milligrams of calcium per day. Teens need about 1,200 milligrams. The pregnant mother needs an additional 400 milligrams per day. To give you an idea of what this means, a cup of milk gives approximately 300 milligrams. An ounce of cheddar cheese has about 200 milligrams. Yogurt has about 400 milligrams. Calcium pills help, but only a little, and may contain contaminants, including arsenic, mercury, and lead. These pills typically contain between 20 and 40 milligrams per capsule.

Nutrients

	Before Pregnancy	During Pregnancy	Breast-Feeding
Folic Acid	400 mg	800	600
Niacin	14 mg	16	18
Protein	46 g	76	66
Riboflavin	1.4 mg	1.7	1.9
Thiamin	1.1 mg	1.4	1.4

Minerals

	Before Pregnancy	During Pregnancy	Breast-Feeding
Calcium	800 mg	1,200	1,200
Iodine	115 mcg	125	150
Iron	18 mg	18+	18
Magnesium	300 mg	450	450
Phosphorus	800 mg	1,200	1,200
Zinc	15 mg	20	25

Vitamins

	Before Pregnancy	During Pregnancy	Breast-Feeding
A (IU)	4,000	5,000	6,000
B_6 (mg)	2	2.5	2.5
B_{12} (mg)	3	4	4
C (mg)	45	60	80
D (IU)	400	400	400
E (IU)	12	15	15

Snacks are fine as long as they aren't heavy in calories with little nutritional value. Nutritious snacks are best, and are good for Mom and baby.

There are also harmful things that Mom can take into her body to watch out for. Keep in mind that everything she takes in also goes to the baby. It's sometimes surprising that the woman who would never dream of slipping a little of her martini into a baby's bottle won't hesitate to go on a weekend drunk.

Heavy drinking has been linked to *fetal alcohol syndrome* (FAS). Deformities, growth problems, and mental retardation can be the result. Although something like an occasional glass of wine is unlikely to cause harm, even a single drink per day has been known to bring on problems with the child's intellect and attention span. Some in the medical profession suggest that Mom not have even one drink while trying to conceive and throughout the pregnancy.

What you do to yourself is your own business (and sometimes the business of the law). Being pregnant is a time to reevaluate those personal choices and "freedoms." You (and she) are no longer affecting only yourself.

Take something as simple as smoking. The smoking mother stands a greatly increased chance of having a premature baby, or one that is undersized. Also increased are the chances of a miscarriage, fetal death, or neonatal death (SIDS—sudden infant death syndrome). The nicotine and carbon monoxide of a cigarette get into the baby quickly, causing constriction of the blood vessels, thus reducing the amount of oxygen and nourishment. There are also indications that the baby of a smoking mother can sustain permanent damage that can make the baby less intelligent and less coordinated.

It doesn't stop there. It's easy to tell Mom to stop smoking, drinking, and whatever while she's pregnant. Don't forget that you're a part of it. For example, your own cigarette smoke is being inhaled by the mother, even if she doesn't light up herself. If both of you smoke, demanding that she quit while you continue can be seen as unfair, whereas if both of you quit, you form your own little support group.

Yet another part of this is chemicals taken in unintentionally. Pesticides are an obvious example. Any number of other agents can also be harmful. Solvents, some art materials, photographic chemicals, hair dye, and cleaning substances are just a few of the things that can bring on consequences. This doesn't mean that Mom has to hide herself away in a sterile environment, just that both of you need to be aware.

Fetal Growth

What's going on inside?

You already know that both the egg and sperm are literally microscopic before conception, and that cell division begins to occur almost immediately after conception. It's a too common misbelief that the growing embryo is little more than a mass of cells. Technically the fertilized egg is called an embryo until it has developed enough to look like a human baby (after which it is called a fetus). This takes just nine weeks. But development occurs earlier.

At twenty-two days the fertilized egg is still barely visible. At thirty-five days the backbone begins to form and the embryo is about one-twelfth inch long and one-sixth inch wide. By the sixth week the head and heart are forming and visible. The embryo is now one-fourth inch long. A week later the embryo has a distinct chest and abdomen. Fingers and toes are forming. Eyes are visible. The embryo at this point is about one-half inch long. In the eighth week, about two months after conception, facial features, including a nose and ears, are present. The new child now weighs about one gram—about the same as a paper clip.

In the ninth week the face is complete. Arms, hands, legs, and feet are formed. The child now looks very much like a miniature version of what you will see when the child is born. Weight has doubled to two grams. It is now called a fetus, rather than an embryo.

By three months, nails appear on the fingers and toes. Genitals are forming. Completely formed eyelids are closed. The arms and legs have begun to move. The child is now about three inches long and about one ounce (thirty grams). This is the end of the first trimester, and in a way is the end of this chapter. By the time those first months are over, living inside her is a living, moving miniature of the child that is to come. Of course, the growth and development don't stop here.

In the second trimester, fine hair has started to grow on the body, including eyebrows and eyelashes. In the fifth month, hair on the head is obvious. By six months, the child is basically fully formed, and may even survive outside the womb. The eyes are open.

By the beginning of the third trimester (at seven months), the unborn stands at least a fifty-fifty chance of survival outside the womb. If there are no complications or health problems, survival rate is above 90 percent. Length will be roughly sixteen inches, with the weight approaching four pounds. In the eighth month the survival rate is more than 90 percent. Weight is just over five pounds.

At term (approximately nine months) the average child weighs seven and one half pounds and is twenty inches long. There will be hair on the head about one inch long. With modern medicine, the chances that the child will survive are more than 99 percent, with most newborn deaths being the result of complications, health problems in either the mother or child, or birth defects. Almost always it is known ahead of time that the pregnancy is in the high-risk category.

Incidentally, the risk of the mother dying in labor or while giving birth is about 1 in 12,500; again, most of these are "high risk." This comes out to be 0.008 percent. It is dramatically lower if the mother is healthy and has done all the right things (taken care of herself, eaten a proper diet, seen the doctor regularly, etc.) during the pregnancy.

What Else Can You Do?

The first trimester is a time of changes and of preparation. Whether this is the first pregnancy for you and/or your wife, or the tenth, there are going to be many surprises in store for both of you. Most will be pleasant. A few may not be.

If you fall for the false notion that the man's job is to get her pregnant and then pay the bills, you're going to miss out on one of the richest experiences of your life. These first months are the time to get involved, and stay involved.

Take this time to learn. You already have this book. There are plenty of others (although almost none are aimed at the father). Mom probably has at least one. Libraries and bookstores will usually have plenty of them.

You probably won't attend a childbirth class this early, but check into it. Find out who is offering what, when, and how much it will cost. You may find that the classes fill up fast. You don't want to be entering the third trimester only to have no openings available in any of the classes.

Mostly, enjoy this time. Be a part of it. Support your wife and try to understand what she is going through. Spend time together. This doesn't have to be about the baby. Sit together and watch a movie on TV. Take a walk. Go out for dinner. Rekindle the romance that brought you together in the first place. In short, develop a closeness between you. This will help to make everything go smoother, and to be more fun.

7

Middle Pregnancy

*T*he second trimester begins in the thirteenth week and ends at the twenty-seventh week. Normally these middle months are the most pleasant part of the pregnancy. Mom's body has adjusted to the flood of hormones and to the changes. Her mind (and hopefully yours as well) has adjusted to the idea of being pregnant, and of eventually being a mother (and father). Yet the due date is still far enough away that this doesn't overshadow things.

As mentioned in the last chapter, Mom often feels fatigued in the first trimester. It's likely that she will again as the birth comes closer. During the second trimester, however, she will probably be more "normal." Usually, if she has felt morning sickness, it fades or disappears in the second trimester. And the discomforts of the third trimester haven't started.

For most, this is the most pleasant part of the pregnancy.

It's a great time for the couple to grow closer. You can truly begin to work together toward what will be one of the most important events in your lives. You're going to be parents in a few more months!

During the second trimester Mom will begin to "show." It will soon become apparent to everyone that she is pregnant. She will start to get attention from others, even total strangers. Yet she hasn't become so large that she feels fat. (Don't rely on this as an absolute. Water retention and other conditions can cause her to *feel* fat.)

During this second trimester you can take care of many of the details. It's not too early to find out about paternity leave at work. The company may not offer one, but it's rare that they won't make accommodations so you can be there when your child is born and at least for a short time after. If they know well enough ahead of time, the arrangements will be easier on everyone.

A related concern may be maternity leave for Mom. This could come up sooner than you think, and will certainly take longer than your own time away from work. During the pregnancy there will probably be days when she doesn't feel well. This is more likely to happen in the first and third trimesters, and particularly toward the end. It's possible that she'll need (and deserve) at least two weeks before delivery and two weeks after. Maybe more—on both sides.

By planning ahead, at least part of this time can be "vacation." It's possible that the rest can be worked out in various ways—*if* you plan ahead. For example, she might be able to work part-time as the due date approaches, then part-time again after a suitable recovery time. These days more and more people are able to work from home, with a more flexible schedule.

In 1993 Congress enacted the Family and Medical Leave Act. This is now a federal law. Its purpose is to guarantee that an employee can take up to twelve weeks off for medical reasons without the danger of losing employment (i.e., it's a violation of federal law for the employer to fire you for this reason). Even assuming that you can afford to take off so much time, the law may or may not apply to you. Certain criteria have to be met. For example, you must have been employed for at least one year, and must have worked at least 1,250 hours in that year.

It might be worthwhile to check with your employer. (The personnel office will know if the law applies and if you qualify.) Also check with your wife's employer, if she works.

Another possibility to consider and discuss is a change in career. This might be the excuse needed for her to leave the job she is in entirely, and to then either stay at home with the child(ren), or to later seek a different job. Be prepared for Mom not wanting to go back to work. Even more, be prepared for her to feel conflict. Both are common. In this you can be a big help by being supportive.

Don't forget some of these same possibilities for yourself. Beyond paternity leave, or lack of it, you might be able to plan your own vacation to be around at this important time. Remember that you can't predict the exact birth date. By planning ahead with your employer, perhaps that vacation can be a little more open-ended. It would be silly to have your vacation time locked in when it wasn't needed, and gone when it was needed. Dropping this kind of situation on the employer at the last minute is unfair. If you plan ahead, in this second trimester, it just might work out well for all concerned.

After the birth, Mom could use some extra help at home. Would it be possible for you to work part-time for a while? Or perhaps work at home?

These are tough questions for both of you. They involve income at a time when you need more of it. They involve changing your lifestyles, possibly in drastic ways. It's for this reason that thinking about it now (or earlier) is so important. What are your options? What can you do about them? In this second trimester you have the time to work together to make these tough decisions, and to plan for them.

If you haven't already selected names, doing so now can be fun. It also gives you plenty of time to pick just the right name. The two of you can talk about it, make lists, change your minds, pick another name. Sometime in the second trimester, your baby will begin to move. This tends to truly cement the idea that you are about to become parents. Now . . . what will we call our baby?

At home, this is a great time to repaint the baby's room. Both of you probably have more energy now than you did during the first trimester (at least Mom does), and more than you'll have in the third trimester. Just as important, if not more so, remodeling now allows plenty of time for the fumes to clear. Finally, preparing the baby's room is another great excuse for working together.

Couples usually decide to attend childbirth classes late into the second trimester. Others prefer to wait until the third. Either way, don't put it off *too* much longer. Remember that few babies are born on the predicted due date. Attending classes in the second trimester prepares you, and also gives time to practice the breathing and relaxing techniques. At very least, the second trimester is a good time to find out about classes and to register.

The Fetus Grows

Growth continues during the second trimester. It increases in some ways but slows in others. Hands and feet have become well formed. The genitals will have started to form by that third month. By the end of the third month the sex difference is obvious (if you could look inside). Nails will have formed on the fingers and toes.

About midway through the fourth month, and midway through the pregnancy, definite fetal movement may be felt (or may not). When either of you notices definite movement of the fetus, make a note of it. (Normally this happens at twenty weeks.) Be sure that the doctor is told at the next regular visit. This information will help to determine the actual age of the child. The predicted delivery date can then be adjusted, if need be.

It's important to remember that no two pregnancies are alike. Usually the mother can feel fetal movement somewhere between the eighteenth and twenty-first weeks. If she doesn't, there is probably no need for concern. Sometimes the baby doesn't begin to move around much until as late as the twenty-sixth week, and it could be even longer before the movements are distinct. Even more common is a baby that doesn't move much, that moves slowly, or that moves gently. Some women think they are having a rumbling in the tummy, such as being hungry, when in fact this is the baby "fluttering."

The baby will begin to have bouts of hiccups, but neither of you is likely to notice this. Remember that the baby isn't breathing yet. All needed oxygen comes to it through the mother's blood supply. The nose, throat, and lungs are filled with fluid at this time. At most the hiccups produce tiny jerks.

By the fifth month the baby will be a little over seven inches long and will weigh about one pound. Fine hair, called *lanugo*, grows. The skin becomes covered with *vernix*, a white coating with a cheeselike texture. This helps to protect the growing baby.

Your child will react to sounds starting in the fifth month. Just what this means is uncertain. Some claim that even this early, the unborn child is learning to recognize the sounds of the parents' voices. You may have some people tell you that arguments or loud noises will permanently mar the child's psyche. Still others say that you can further influence the unborn, depending on the kinds of sounds it hears. (One story says that gentle music causes a gentle child, while fast music brings a nervous child.)

Two thirds of the way through the pregnancy—at six months—the eyes may open. Weight is up to about three pounds. If born, the baby stands about a 50 percent chance of survival, although complications of some kind are almost certain. From this point on, the chances of survival grow steadily.

Over the next three months, your baby will complete development. It will put on roughly another five pounds and grow another nine or ten inches in length. If Mom hasn't already started to "show," she will in the third trimester.

Both her body and the baby's are in for a lot more changes.

Changes in Mom

Actually, Mom has been going through a number of changes. Many of them are rather subtle during the second trimester. Others are more obvious, and can sometimes be almost overwhelming. Despite the many changes you're likely to notice, chances are very good that everything is perfectly normal. Your job is simply to be aware.

Increased appetite is normal. She's eating for two. During the second trimester the fetus inside grows from about an ounce to three pounds. Supportive tissue is also needed. The amniotic sac grows and fills with fluid. By nature, Mom's body also puts on more fat.

On the average, the newborn weighs about seven and a half pounds. Also on the average, Mom will gain almost three times this much during the pregnancy. Most of this will come in the last trimester, but weight gain in the second trimester is likely to be noticeable. To keep track of it, Mom will be weighed at each visit to the doctor. She should be gaining weight—not too much, and not too little.

Food cravings are also normal. Often this is an indication of a dietary need. Even if Mom is doing most or all of the cooking, you can help make sure that both of you (particularly she) are getting a balanced diet.

It's possible that the doctor should be informed, and he should definitely be informed if the cravings are powerful or strange. Supplements may be prescribed. (DO NOT undertake this on your own.)

The classic craving is for pickles and ice cream. Actually this is rare. Cravings of this sort are also usually harmless. Unusual cravings include the desire to eat things such as dirt or even laundry detergent. Such bizarre cravings should be brought to the attention of the doctor at the next visit. If Mom gives in, more immediate action needs to be taken.

Increasing backaches are normal. Most of the time it's due to a softening of the pelvic muscles, growth of the amniotic sac and fetus, and a shifting of the center of gravity. The last can cause a change in posture, which in turn puts a strain on the spine and lower back.

Also normal are abdominal pains and muscle cramping. As the amniotic sac expands, organs are pushed aside. Muscles and ligaments are stretched. Mom might even feel that she is having contractions (which is possible).

Mild and irregular pains such as these are normal and to be expected. They should be mentioned to the doctor, but probably are not a cause for concern. At the same time, these can be early warning signs of serious trouble. For example, they might be a warning of an ectopic pregnancy (see "Other Changes" in Chapter Six).

Possibly related is *diastasis*. This means that the muscles across the tummy, called the *rectus abdominis* muscles, have separated. The uterus can protrude from beneath. The separation can also cause backache. In most cases, this doesn't cause a big problem. Chances are good that the muscles will knit together again after the birth. Assuming that Mom attends her regular appointments with the doctor, he'll know soon if this has happened, and if it will cause a problem.

Leg cramps are fairly common. These can be caused by

a lack of calcium in the diet, by the expanding uterus pinching nerves, or even by simple fatigue. Although these should
be mentioned to the doctor, they probably do not indicate
anything serious. You can help by watching the diet, and
with foot and leg massage. Don't forget the value of taking
on a few more of the household chores.

Digestive problems are also common. Keep in mind, the
uterus is growing and expanding. Other organs, such as the
stomach, are being squeezed. At the same time, hormones
are suppressing the digestive system. This can cause indigestion, heartburn, and constipation. In most cases, none are of
great concern unless they are severe, prolonged, or are accompanied by other symptoms. The two main cautions are
to (as always) keep the doctor informed, and never try to treat
the symptoms yourselves. Even a simple over-the-counter
antacid is to be avoided without the doctor's recommendation.

With this may, and probably will, come an increased
need for her to urinate. This is almost certain to increase in
the third trimester. The cause is much the same as for digestive problems. Her system is changing while the bladder is
being squeezed into a smaller space. It might get frustrating
if the two of you are out shopping and she needs to find a
rest room so often. It's just part of being pregnant.

Expect changes in the skin. Darkening of the nipples,
armpits, thighs, and perineum are common. The linea nigra
is likely to become more pronounced.

Moles and freckles may develop. Those she already has
might darken or grow larger. All this is normal. Even so, it
warrants a mention to the doctor. This becomes especially
important if the mole is painful or seems infected. Increased
acne may also occur, although it tends to begin to clear after
the fourth or fifth month. Mom should not use any medication for this, including topical creams and ointments, other
than what the doctor prescribes.

Shortness of breath is fairly common, but needs watching. It's very common for her to begin snoring as the pregnancy progresses. As the fetus grows, pressure is being applied in all directions, including against the lungs and diaphragm. This can cause some difficulty in breathing. It shouldn't be severe. If it is, contact the doctor.

Another common symptom is a pounding heart, or the heart skipping a beat now and then. Once again, there is probably no cause for concern, but the doctor needs to be told. This becomes more important, possibly critical, if the pounding heart comes with a shortness of breath, and possibly critical if it's also accompanied by headaches and/or dizziness.

One possibly frightening symptom might be an increase in nosebleeds and bleeding gums. During pregnancy, estrogen levels increase, as does the supply of blood. The estrogen can cause the gums to soften. That can cause the bleeding. Along with this comes an increase in tooth decay.

It will help if Mom gets a thorough checkup from a dentist before the pregnancy. If she goes *during* the pregnancy, she should advise the dentist that she is pregnant. The reason is because anesthetics and some kinds of dental work or surgery can affect Mom, and the fetus. If the dentist says that a procedure is needed, Mom should consult with her obstetrician to be sure that the procedure will be safe.

Mom should brush and floss after every meal. She should also avoid sugary foods or any foods that cause plaque.

Another frightening possible occurrence is called an umbilical hernia. The outer sign is a protruding belly button. The doctor should be told—although he'll notice anyway— but this kind of hernia is rarely a problem. It will probably correct itself after the birth.

Problems and Warnings

One of the terrible things that can happen is a *miscarriage*, more accurately called *spontaneous abortion*. If this happens early in the first trimester, it's possible that no one will know. Even later in the first trimester, and after the pregnancy is confirmed, a miscarriage is more easily accepted for what it usually is—a pregnancy that didn't quite "take."

By the second trimester, the parents usually know that there is a pregnancy, and that the fetus is becoming well formed. The emotions stirred by the loss tend to be stronger. Of course, these increase even more in the third trimester, but so do the chances that the child can be saved.

The turning point is usually considered to be the twenty-fourth week, late in the second trimester. Before the twenty-third week, there is little chance for the fetus to survive. By that magical twenty-fourth week, the chances are fifty-fifty. Instead of *miscarriage* or *spontaneous abortion*, the situation begins to be called *preterm birth*. This topic will be covered in more depth in the next chapter (it's more likely to happen in the third trimester) and in Chapter Eleven. For now, be aware of the potential warning signs.

Even a slight vaginal discharge can send many will-be-parents into a panic. Although, once again, you should never try self-diagnosis, most such vaginal discharges are either normal or represent no danger. For example, a thin, clear-to-white discharge could be hormonal in cause, or might be the indication of a vaginal infection. This needs medical attention, but is no reason to panic. Of greater concern is a discharge that is gray or green, and particularly if it is tinged with blood (or has a pinkish color, perhaps due to blood).

Chances are good that any of these symptoms is a sign of a treatable infection, but if there is color, foaminess, or strong odor, the doctor should be contacted quickly. The same is true if Mom begins to have contractions. More than five contractions in an hour warrants an immediate call to the doctor. If the discharge has appreciable volume, get to the emergency room immediately.

The risks increase if Mom has had a miscarriage or abortion before, if she is carrying more than one child, or if she has suffered from a serious illness or infection during the pregnancy.

About 25 percent of all miscarriages are brought on by a condition called *cervical incompetence*. This simply means that the cervix begins to soften and dilate too early. It is usually caused by a weakness of the cervix. As the fetus grows, and the uterus with it, pressure on the already weak cervix increases. It becomes unable to hold the child.

If diagnosed properly and early, the condition can often be taken care of with a surgical procedure called *cerclage*. There are actually several such methods. The doctor(s) will determine which is best in her case. It is usually performed before the eighteenth week of the pregnancy.

Also in order is increased rest. For some women this can even mean being confined to bed. If that sounds like fun, and time off with no cares, think again. After just a few days, it's not only boring, it's hard on the body.

Preeclampsia is high blood pressure induced by pregnancy. It affects about 7 percent of all pregnant women, with most of these being in their first pregnancy. Fortunately, it is usually fairly mild and easily treatable. It's rare in the early weeks of pregnancy and generally develops after the twentieth week, but more commonly after the twenty-eighth week. If untreated, it presents a threat to both the mother and baby. In very serious cases, it can even be fatal. For both!

With most women, the onset of preeclampsia goes unnoticed. There are no outward symptoms. Mom's blood pressure will be taken at each visit to the doctor. This way preeclampsia can be caught early—before it becomes eclampsia (*very* high blood pressure). Even with preeclampsia, the blood supply to the placenta, and thus to the growing baby, is reduced. This can affect fetal growth. With eclampsia, the blood supply may be closed off completely!

There are often no outward symptoms. By the time there are, preeclampsia has already set in. As is so often the case, almost every symptom has alternate explanations. For example, preeclampsia can cause edema, especially in the hands and face. So can water retention, which might be caused by too much salt in the diet. Headaches and changes in eyesight are other symptoms of preeclampsia—but can also be from perfectly ordinary causes.

A more serious symptom is a sudden gain in weight. If Mom gains more than two pounds in a week, or six pounds in a month, something is wrong. The baby doesn't grow that fast, nor does Mom. This much weight gain almost certainly comes from a sudden retention of fluids.

Treatment of mild preeclampsia will probably be a change in diet, and perhaps some changes in lifestyle. The doctor may suggest bed rest, and is also likely to tell Mom to lie on her left side, or sometimes the right side, to allow a better flow of blood to the placenta. Depending on the severity, hospitalization might be required. It's even possible that labor will have to be induced, or the baby removed via C-section.

The Doctors

Most pregnancies run a standard routine through the second trimester. Visits to the doctor, after the first visit to determine pregnancy, usually take place about every three weeks. This will continue probably into the eighth month. The visits will then become closer.

Make it a point to go to the exams at least during the second trimester. There really isn't much to them. Mom comes in, gives the nurse a urine sample, and is weighed. Blood pressure is taken. If needed, a blood sample will be drawn for testing.

In the exam room she lifts her shirt over her tummy. The doctor feels to determine growth and placement. The baby's heartbeat is checked, usually with a Doppler probe. (Both of you will be able to listen—and hear the beat of your baby's heart.) Mom will be asked if she has any complaints or questions. Assuming all is normal and well, the exam will last no more than ten to fifteen minutes.

A glucose tolerance test may be taken. *Gestational diabetes* is a fairly common occurrence. Caught early and treated, it rarely causes problems. Left alone, it can bring on all sorts of troubles, particularly for the fetus. The least of this is called *macrosomia*, which means that the child is overweight. The usual dividing line is at nine and three-fourths pounds. Delivery of the large baby is going to be more difficult, which increases the possibility of injury to both the child and mother.

The risk is higher for women over thirty, and certainly for women who come from families with a history of diabetes. Women who are overweight going into the pregnancy are also at a higher risk. Even so, about half of all cases of gestational diabetes are in women who don't fit into any category. It's because of this that many doctors routinely watch the glucose level. It's also very common for the doctor to order a more complex glucose tolerance screening.

The most common time for this test is between twenty-four and twenty-eight weeks. Some doctors order the test immediately after the initial exam. Some will want it repeated several times during the pregnancy, especially if Mom falls into one of the higher-risk categories.

The test itself is very simple. Mom will be given a glucose drink. After an hour, blood is taken and tested. Most of the time, everything is just fine. In about 15 percent of the cases, the first test will show an abnormal level of glucose. If so, a second test is given.

For this, Mom is told to not eat anything until the next day. Again she is given a glucose drink and a blood sample is taken. Most will "pass" this second test. Either way, a closer monitoring of glucose levels will probably be ordered.

This is one of the reasons that the urine is tested each

time Mom goes in. A part of it is to test the glucose level. This test isn't as complete or certain but provides a quick and easy method for monitoring the possible onset of diabetes. It is also helpful for spotting other potential health problems, including infections and preeclampsia.

Anemia is another fairly common problem. It affects about 20 percent of all pregnant women. Mom's blood volume will increase by about 50 percent during the pregnancy. This can cause iron deficiency, which can bring on anemia. Although anemia sets in usually after the twentieth week, it's not unusual for the doctor to test for it earlier.

A woman normally needs about twice as much iron as a man. (Before puberty and after menopause, her need is the same as for the male.) The need for iron doubles during pregnancy. Usually this can be taken care of with minor changes in diet or with vitamin/mineral supplements. Unfortunately, iron supplements tend to cause nausea.

Insufficient folic acid can also cause anemia. Folic acid (a part of the vitamin B complex) is important in the production of red blood cells. As the amount of blood increases, more and more red blood cells are needed, which in turn means more folic acid is needed. Good natural sources are green vegetables, liver, and yeast.

Alpha-fetoprotein levels in the blood may be tested. This substance is given off by the growing fetus. If the level is too high, it could indicate a neural tube defect. A level that is too low could mean Down's syndrome. Either way, additional testing will be done to verify the diagnosis.

Various other tests may also be performed. It's important for the doctor, and for both of you, to spot potential problems early. Not only is treatment easier, the sooner treatment begins, the less damage will be caused. Because many of the tests are suggested by symptoms, it's important that Mom be open and honest with the doctor. For example, if she has been having headaches, the doctor won't know unless she tells him.

What Can You Do?

As the birth approaches, there will be more and more changes in and around your home. Attention shifts increasingly toward Mom. This is as it should be, but it's not unusual for the father to feel left out. An accessory. If you don't get those feelings, great! If you do, realize that they are quite common, and in many ways are justifiable.

Mom *does* come first. This doesn't mean that your role isn't important. It's going to be even more important from now on.

During the second trimester everything will probably flow smoothly, with few pregnancy-related complaints. For most, it's the best period. Both of you are adjusting to the situation, and to the fact that a new life is about to join your own. The first trimester is over, and things tend to be more "settled in." The third trimester, in which Mom may have nearly constant physical complaints, hasn't started.

It can be a great time, during which the two of you have the opportunity to become even more close. It's a time for planning and preparing. If all goes as it usually does, the second trimester will be a time of growth—not just for the fetus but for both of you.

It's also a time to remain aware. Most problems come either in the first or third trimesters, but some of the potential dangers can be spotted and treated in the second. If caught soon enough, the danger can be minimized, or done away with completely. For example, conditions such as preeclampsia might show up. If it's caught and treated, the risks can be minimized. Ignored, the condition can escalate to the point of becoming fatal.

Be aware of what Mom is experiencing. Listen to her complaints. Help her keep a list of complaints and questions to bring to the doctor. Encourage her to be honest with the doctor, not secretive. (Don't forget to encourage her to keep each and every appointment!)

By the second trimester, your diets should already be well balanced. If not, don't wait any longer! You should also have the doctors and hospital well on the way to being paid off. If you're not already attending a childbirth class, arrange for one.

Most of all, don't miss the opportunities this trimester offers. The exams are more routine rather than intimate. You can attend without embarrassing Mom or yourself. You can listen to the heartbeat of your child for the first time. If ultrasound is used, you might even get to see the little rascal.

Make use of this period. Enjoy it.

Enjoy it together!

8

The Last Months

*T*he third trimester begins at week twenty-eight and goes to term. The average is thirty-eight gestational (since conception) weeks, or forty weeks from her last period before conception. This "standard," however is accurate only 5 percent of the time. A week before or after is quite common. Two weeks isn't unusual—although the doctor will probably consider inducing labor if Mom is more than two weeks overdue.

By the beginning of this last trimester, the baby has already reached the point of development at which it is likely to survive. (As mentioned in the last chapter, the critical turning point is twenty-four weeks.) Everything is in place. The last trimester is more one of growth and maturation. Your baby will also develop an important layer of fat.

You can expect Mom to become increasingly uncomfortable. Some of the problems of the first and second trimesters will return, and are likely to become worse. New complaints will begin. The backaches, swollen ankles, shortness of breath, and much more are likely to *strike with a vengeance*! Other problems, such as preeclampsia (high blood pressure) and gestational diabetes, can become worse, or may show up for the first time.

During those first two trimesters, there hasn't been a lot you could actually do. In this final trimester, Mom needs you. With your help, this trimester can be much more pleasant for her—and for both of you. Relaxing together in the evening while you rub her feet and her back, talking about the baby that will soon be yours, can develop memories you will never forget. This kind of support will help Mom directly and immediately, and in the longer term can help to create a bond between you that can carry you through any rough times.

"I'm So Fat!"

Expect to hear this. Often! No matter how many times you try to remind Mom that she's not fat, she's pregnant, it won't seem to do much good. Just how you express this depends largely on her personality, and on the circumstances.

During the pregnancy Mom will usually put on between twenty and twenty-five pounds. Her digestive system will change. Fluid retention is common, causing a feeling of being bloated. She'll have aches and pains, a loss of balance, and many other problems. It will be pretty obvious that Mom has put on weight. What counts just as much, or more, is that she often *feels* fat.

Sometimes verbal reassurance is enough, but it should be coupled with other signs of affection and caring. This isn't a gender thing. All of us, men and women, enjoy the feeling of having someone care, who finds us attractive. Words alone aren't always enough. In fact, there are times when, as the old expression goes, action speaks louder than words. In both directions!

Cheryl began gaining weight. Her husband, Larry, trying to show his concern, monitored her diet religiously. Because of her physical complaints, and his fear of injuring her or the baby, he stopped having sex with her. Each night he would lovingly (to him) rub her feet and legs. Each time she would mention how fat she was getting, he'd pass it off with, "You're not fat, honey, you're pregnant!"

The words were there. So were some of the right actions. Along with them came actions that strengthened her worry that she was no longer attractive to him. His watching her diet gave her the notion that even though he was *saying* she wasn't fat, it was a lie. Why would he be so involved in every morsel she ate if he really meant it? Also, to her, avoiding her sexually was "positive proof" that he no longer found her attractive.

It can be tricky finding the correct solutions, and virtually impossible to find those solutions each and every time. What if Larry had shown no interest in his wife's diet? What if he made moves to have sex on a regular basis?

You *should* become involved if Mom is truly putting on *too* much weight. This can be detrimental to her and to the baby. The same is true if the cravings she has become abnormal (such as wanting to eat laundry detergent or dirt).

Everything becomes easier if it starts early, and if you participate. Instead of munching salty, greasy potato chips, try to become accustomed to fresh vegetables or apple slices.

More Changes

The final trimester is not comfortable for Mom. The morning sickness that may have affected her in the first trimester is probably gone. (If she does suffer from nausea or dizziness, inform the doctor immediately!) But the closer she comes to term, the more uncomfortable she is going to be. In many ways. In other ways, she can become more comfortable.

Usually about a month before the birth, the baby "drops." By the thirtieth week, the baby will tend to settle in the head-down position. By the thirty-sixth week, the head is usually nestled into the pelvic region. (For a woman who has had other babies, it may not happen until the onset of labor.) This is called *lightening,* which describes the feeling well. The baby moves lower, and settles its head in the pelvis. As the baby moves down, pressure on the lungs and other organs is reduced. Mom can breathe almost normally again. At the same time, however, pressure increases elsewhere.

Frequent urination increases, sometimes to the point of causing an accident. Due to pressure and distortion of the bladder and urethra, and the resulting difficulty in emptying the bladder, bladder infections are more common. Quite often this is spotted with the urine test during the regular visits to the doctor. It's another reason why those visits come more often at the end, and why it's so important for Mom to keep every appointment.

Many women experience a swelling of the legs, ankles, and feet throughout the third trimester. This often increases as full term approaches. Pressure of the fetus on the blood vessels makes circulation to the legs more difficult. This can cause the lower extremities to fill with fluid.

If it's severe, the doctor should be notified, especially if the swelling comes up quickly. In most cases, massage can relieve the condition. (If the swelling is severe, ask the doctor first. In a few rare cases, massage can be detrimental.) Begin at the toes and massage toward the heart. The goal is to help move the trapped fluids back up into the body. (See the Appendix on "Massage.")

There can be many causes of the backache Mom is likely to experience. Several of these have been discussed earlier because that's when those causes (e.g., ectopic pregnancy) occur. By the third trimester, although backache can be brought on by something serious, it usually has to do with two primary factors.

The easiest to understand is the change in the center of balance. Becoming more and more popular is a device that Dad can put on to get the feel of what it's like to be pregnant, with all that weight low and in front. While being a good demonstration in general, it doesn't allow for the gradual adjustment to the change. Mom has had months to adjust as the fetus grows. Such a device suddenly strapped to a person allows no gradual period of adjustment.

That doesn't make Mom's lack of balance any less real, however. Carrying an additional twenty-five pounds or so, twenty-four hours a day, every day, can make the lower back sore.

The uterus is supported by round ligaments. Especially toward the end of the pregnancy, these are stretched and strained. Sometimes the pangs caused by this can be severe enough to cause Mom to think she is going into labor, or that she has appendicitis.

Upper abdominal pains can also lead Mom to think she is going into premature labor or has some other dread medical problem. These often feel much like a charley horse. One of the more common causes is pressure against the liver and other organs by the growing fetus. It's also possible that the abdominal muscles have separated. For both, there won't be much the doctor can do. Even so, the doctor needs to know, just in case the cause is something more serious, but chances are the only cure is for the baby to be born, and for Mom to have a suitable time to recover and heal.

Don't take her claims and fears lightly. She could be right! Chances are everything is fine. The only one qualified to make the diagnosis is the doctor.

Constipation and Hemorrhoids

Another common problem that tends to increase in the final trimester is constipation. As mentioned before in this book, the entire digestive system changes during pregnancy. This can bring on indigestion and nausea. Progesterone causes the bowel to become more relaxed. Pressure from the growing fetus squeezes the bowel. The combination brings on constipation. This is most common late in the pregnancy because that's when the fetus is largest.

It has been said a number of times in this book—a sound, balanced diet that begins even before the pregnancy really helps to minimize, and even eliminate, many of the problems and discomforts. Reduced salt can help reduce edema. Plenty of fresh fruit and vegetables, and increased fiber, can help constipation.

Also as you've read many times here, never self-prescribe. Without the doctor's okay, Mom shouldn't use even over-the-counter antacids, laxatives, or anything else. Not even aspirin!

A fairly common treatment for constipation is mineral oil. It's fairly gentle, has no chemicals that can affect the baby (hopefully), but brings with it another kind of problem. Mineral oil can block absorption of fat-soluble vitamins. Among these are A, D, and E. Mom and the baby need all of these. Using mineral oil to relieve constipation can result in Mom not getting enough of these essential vitamins.

Related to constipation are hemorrhoids. It's unusual for a woman to not get hemorrhoids—if not late in the pregnancy, then almost certainly during birthing. The fetus presses against the anorectal veins. This can trap fluids in the lower extremities, and also increases the chances of hemorrhoids.

If Mom strains too hard, due to constipation (or birthing),

hemorrhoids can result. These rarely cause a major problem, but can be uncomfortable or painful. There is also the possibility of a local infection, made worse because wiping can also be painful. This leaves the area less clean.

The first step is, again, a good diet that is high in fiber. You can help by bringing Mom a plate of sliced apples as a snack, instead of chocolates. (Better yet, bring enough for both of you, and share them while you give her a tender foot rub.) The doctor may, or may not, prescribe a stool softener to help relieve the constipation, and to reduce Mom's urge, and need, to push so hard.

To help keep the tender area clean, Mom could wash the area rather than wipe. A shower head on a long hose works well for this. It makes it easy to direct the flow of water right to where it is needed. This not only keeps the area clean, it can provide some relief in itself.

Another solution is to use treated wipes, available in containers or packets. They provide soothing coolness while cleaning the area.

Just as progesterone relaxes the bowel, it relaxes the fleshy valve to the stomach. This brings us back to overall changes in the digestive system, and pressure put on the organs by the growing fetus. By now this combination should sound quite familiar. This time it causes not only indigestion but heartburn. Food and the natural acids that occur in the stomach can be squeezed from the stomach through the relaxed valve and into the esophagus.

The best cure is a change in diet. Mom should avoid foods that are greasy, acidic, spicy, or hard to digest. The list would include coffee, chocolate, cabbage, beans, and much more. It also helps if Mom eats a number of small meals instead of a few larger ("regular") meals. Teas made of peppermint or chamomile can provide some relief.

Other Discomforts and Fears

Some get the sensation of heartburn and think that the best way for quick relief is to lie down. Just the opposite is true. At least a part of the cause is that relaxed stomach valve. By lying down, more of what causes the sensation can leak upward out of the stomach. Standing or sitting allows gravity to help.

Heartburn, need to urinate, cramps, muscle spasms, and more all contribute in robbing Mom of her much-needed sleep. In the second trimester both of you were probably aching for the baby to move, and then spent the next couple of months being thrilled over each movement. Toward the end, some of the thrill is gone, at least for Mom. It can be like having a boxer living inside, ready to pound on your organs.

Try to imagine it. Your bladder is already squeezed so it doesn't hold much, and the urethra is compressed, which makes it difficult to urinate. Then junior inside lays a solid left to the bladder. Or maybe he gives a front kick to the diaphragm.

Mom is uncomfortable at best. Baby is pounding and kicking on her. The internal organs are being moved, squeezed, and punched. Hormones are shifting again. Psychologically Mom knows that the birthing is coming very soon. She may have been able to relax during the second trimester, but now the "real thing" is close at hand. She feels bloated, and as though she no longer has control of her own body. She's worried about the baby, and about herself. She may feel concerned that you no longer find her attractive (and never will again—although she knows better).

The result is that Mom may begin to have unusual, frightening, or weird dreams. Some will be about the baby or the birthing. At times it will be as though all her deep fears have been released. A dream might show her giving birth to an animal or monster. Very common are dreams in which Mom finds herself lost in a deep tunnel, or caught on a voyage and not knowing where she is.

While awake, she is likely to become more and more preoccupied with the birthing, and the near future in general. You could find her trying to correct every "fault" you have. Making it more frustrating, blended in might be memory loss. One day she might *demand* that you get off your lazy duff and paint the kitchen blue, and the next day yell at you because it isn't yellow.

Bear in mind that such an extreme is rare. If you've developed a closeness during the first and second trimesters, in which you work together as a team, the third trimester will be easier for both of you. That closeness, and the sense of truly being "in this together," will carry you through almost anything.

Knowledge is another great weapon. Birth is painful and unpredictable. As you talk (and mostly listen), don't avoid the unpleasant possibilities. A C-section might be needed, or something else might go wrong. But rather than dwell on the negative, concentrate on the positive. Chances are good that everything will be fine—that if there are complications, the doctor and hospital can handle it. Despite the "dangers of pregnancy" cited by some, these days the chances of serious trouble the medical field can't handle are very small.

Mom might be determined to have a "natural" childbirth. This is fine, but she also needs to know that if an anesthetic is needed, or even wanted, that's okay, too. It's one thing to imagine the ideal birthing, and quite another to go through it. Even the mother of several children, with each of the previous being an "easy birth," might find this one more difficult.

First-time mothers in particular have the fear of embarrassment. There is the obvious embarrassment of the position she has to be in to give birth. Complicating this, it's not that unusual for the mother to "relieve herself" during the birth.

The nurses are trained for this, and will often clean things up before either of you realize it has happened. Knowing this can help reduce the embarrassment a little, but can also compound it.

"Am I going to pee all over the doctor?" is not a pleasant doubt. The thought of soiling the table with a more solid mess can be even more disconcerting.

More than a few women interviewed said that they were concerned that they might cuss or shout things at the doctor and husband that they really didn't mean. There are even worries about having bad breath, and how you, the father, won't want to be near. Even if your own mate doesn't express this, she might possibly be worried about it.

Much of this can be taken care of if you've been there all along. The concern, caring, and love you've shown during the previous months let her know in a way mere words can't. Through those actions you've told her that you're there for her, no matter what.

Baby's Final Stages of Growth

At the beginning of the third trimester, your baby weighed about two to three pounds and was roughly about a foot in length. Over the next few months, the child will grow to full weight and length. He or she will gain roughly five to six more pounds, and almost double in length.

As stated in the last chapter, week twenty-four marks the point at which the fetus stands a chance of survival outside the womb. By the third trimester, another four weeks have passed. Survival rate has increased (it's already about 90 percent) and will continue to do so.

Basic development is already complete. Now the organs and tissues will grow and mature. Three of the more important are the lungs, digestive system, and body fat. All three are critical to survival but are still immature during at least the first part of the third trimester.

During the third trimester, the child seems to be practicing for life. Movements increase both in number and intensity. You'll be able to feel those movements easily by putting your hand on her tummy. Mom will be feeling them too—sometimes uncomfortably so.

What surprises many people is that the baby sucks his thumb during this trimester, as though preparing to nurse. It is believed that this is an early sign of the rooting reflex. This reflex causes the baby to turn its face toward whatever touches it. In the womb the baby is moving around. At times the thumb will bump into the baby's cheek. Your child will turn his head and begin to suckle.

As body fat develops, the skin becomes smoother and thicker. There are fewer wrinkles. The fine layer of hair (lanugo) begins to disappear.

The lungs begin to develop surfactant. This protein allows them to function correctly. Until this happens, the baby probably won't be able to survive outside the womb, even with a mechanical respirator. During the sixth month, the baby has developed enough surfactant to stand a good chance of survival.

By the seventh month the central nervous system has developed far enough to be able to control the baby's body temperature. During the eighth month, more fat grows under the skin, and the bones harden (except for the skull). The ninth month completes the growth and development. Your baby is ready to come into the world.

Premature Birth

A baby born before the thirty-seventh week is said to be premature, or preterm. In the past this was a frightening time for the parents. Today infants as young as twenty-four or twenty-five weeks stand a good chance of survival. (Sadly, those born before the twenty-third week rarely survive.) Not only do we have the technology to sustain life in the preemie, there is technology available to slow or stop labor. Sometimes the delay of just a few days can make all the difference. There are even medications that help the baby's lungs to mature at a faster rate, which can greatly increase the chances of survival.

About 6 percent of whites experience a severely preterm birth. For blacks the rate is about double. No one knows why. Nor are all the reasons for prematurity understood. For all races, most preterm babies are born close to term and are in little danger.

In other words, the risk of having a preterm baby is fairly low, and the chances of Mom and the baby coming through it successfully are quite high. The situation is further improved if you (both of you) pay attention to danger signs and then do something about them.

A woman who has had a premature birthing before is at a higher risk. Other risk factors include certain medical conditions and illnesses. Once again, it's critical that Mom, and you, be totally honest with the doctor.

At the same time, realize that with a normal pregnancy, physical activity, including sex, does *not* bring on a premature birth. Nor does eating hot or spicy food, seeing a scary movie, a lightning storm, or listening to loud music.

All of these things might cause other problems, however. Some conditions, cervical incompetence, for example, require bed rest. Surgery might help the situation, but the doctor is almost certain to prescribe rest, little or no physical activity, and likely little or no sexual activity.

Cramps or abdominal pains can be an indication of a problem. A twinge now and then is no reason to panic, but deserves mention to the doctor. If it's prolonged or regular, don't wait. Let the doctor know immediately (especially if there are more than five cramps in an hour). The same is true if Mom is feeling pressure in the pelvic region. Vaginal discharge, especially if it has a reddish color, requires immediate attention by a physician.

Even diarrhea or frequent urination are potential symptoms that she is about to give birth prematurely. Like most of the other symptoms, these could also have perfectly normal explanations. The point is that the two of you shouldn't be the ones making the diagnosis.

This applies in both directions. Don't assume that a symptom means something—but don't assume that it *doesn't* mean something. Your best guide is to pay attention throughout the pregnancy. You are looking for changes, especially drastic or sudden ones. Once again this stresses the importance of being a part of everything, and of being aware.

If she goes into labor early, and the doctor already knows the symptoms that have been occurring, the situation can be better controlled. An exam may be needed. A sonogram can be used to help determine the condition. A pelvic exam will show if the cervix is dilating and effacing (expanding and softening—signs of an impending birth).

It's also possible that the doctor will purposely induce labor early. This isn't a time to panic, either. Sometimes the best chance for the baby and the mother comes from inducing an early birthing.

Gestational Diabetes

This topic has been mentioned before. Because of its importance, and because the onset is most likely in the third trimester, it warrants further discussion.

The doctor may or may not order a glucose test early in the pregnancy. It's more likely to be performed at the beginning of the third trimester. Even then, the regular urine tests may be sufficient to indicate that the test may be needed, and likewise that it may not be needed.

Only about 5 percent of all pregnant women get gestational diabetes severely enough to cause concern. That concern, however, is very real.

It is believed that gestational diabetes is triggered mainly by hormones. This causes an increase in the glucose level in the blood. The pancreas normally responds by producing more insulin, but if this doesn't happen, the baby's pancreas will begin to produce more. The problem is that in the fetus, insulin acts as a growth stimulant. An increased insulin level in the baby can cause it to grow too quickly, and too large (macrosomia).

The high level of glucose in the blood can cause other problems. It affects the baby's heart, lungs, and nervous system. This can cause the newborn to have difficulty breathing. This is called respiratory distress syndrome (RDS).

If the condition has caused the baby's pancreas to produce more insulin, it will continue after the baby is born. Now the baby has far too much insulin, which will cause the baby to have low blood sugar. Among other things, if this situation is untreated, brain damage may result.

Although gestational diabetes can affect any woman, it happens more often with women who are overweight, who are already diabetic, and who have had a previous baby that weighed over ten pounds. There also seems to be an increased risk for women over thirty.

The doctor will be checking for this condition. At home, watch for symptoms of increased hunger and thirst, increased urination, or spells of weakness. Remember that each of these symptoms can have other causes, but they should be mentioned to the doctor, just in case. If caught early, treatment is much easier, and damage to Mom or the baby less likely.

Treatment is usually handled by changes in the diet. The doctor may also suggest more regular glucose level monitoring. It's unlikely, but possible, that you'll be asked to do this daily at home. For this, you will probably use a special testing device. A sterile needle pricks the end of the finger. A drop of blood is placed on a test strip, which is then inserted into the device. Within seconds it provides a readout.

Chances are good that the condition can be controlled. If not, the doctor may decide to induce an early labor.

In virtually every case, the diabetes disappears shortly after the birth. However, about half of the women who suffer gestational diabetes will develop permanent diabetes within ten years. For this reason, the doctor may recommend continued dietary control and regular glucose monitoring for Mom.

Nobody completely understands why some women develop diabetes. Indications are that a balanced diet after the birth can minimize, or even eliminate, the chances of it returning. In any case, although monitoring her blood sugar won't prevent or reduce the diabetes, it will let you know when to begin any needed treatments.

Fetal Presentation

The doctor has been checking fetal growth throughout the pregnancy. This is why he feels Mom's tummy at each exam. In the third trimester this becomes both easier and more important. Toward the end he will also be checking the fetal position (presentation).

The majority of babies settle in the head-down position. Ideally the top of the baby's head will be down, and the chin tucked, with the arms and legs crossed. Occasionally the head will be tilted forward, called the brow presentation. In a face presentation, the head is tilted so far that the face of the baby is trying to come out first. The first is normal. The other two (brow and face) could force a C-section.

Sometimes the baby is breech, which means that the bottom is down and the head up. This almost always causes a difficult birth that often ends up with a C-section. A frank breech has the butt down with the legs folded up by the baby's head. It will be rough, but a vaginal birth is possible. Footling breech has a foot coming first. Complete breech has both legs down and folded in a lotus position. Both require a C-section.

The worst position is transverse, with the baby sideways in the womb, perhaps with a shoulder first. Unless the baby can be turned, a C-section is the only option.

Late in the third trimester, usually in the thirty-seventh and thirty-eighth weeks, if the baby is in a potential danger-ous position, the attempt may be made to turn the baby. The process is called *external version*. Commonly, a drug is given to relax the uterus. Massage is then used to reposition the baby. Sometimes it works. Other times the baby will merely flip back around.

This topic will be dealt with in more detail in Chapter Eleven. For now, yet another important reason for Mom to attend each examination is to determine how the baby is positioned. It's possible that a mispresentation can be cor-rected.

What Can You Do?

Your role has been important since even before the con-ception. In the third trimester, through the birthing, and ac-tually from now on, that importance grows. At least it does if you let it. Some kinds of participation are limited. Others may be denied to you. What counts more is that you partic-ipate in every way possible.

When asked what the father could do, almost every woman interviewed responded immediately and loudly with, "Give me a foot rub every night!" (Or a back rub.) This helps relieve some of her aches and pains. Just as important, and for both of you, it provides a time to develop a special closeness.

Some prefer watching a movie. Others like music. In my own case my wife and I spent almost every evening with a fire in the fireplace, and just talking together. What you do depends on your own lifestyle.

Make it a point to spend time together. Any sacrifice you have to make for this time will be well worth it. It can be fun shopping together for the new crib, or painting the baby's room. Even the more mundane things like grocery shopping can be rewarding. And of course, whenever possible, attend the doctor's exam. Listen to the beat of your baby's heart. Attend childbirth classes together.

During this third trimester and for a few weeks after the birth, one of the best things you can do is give Mom special treatment. If she likes flowers, bring her flowers now and then. Even more meaningful is to help around the house. Cook the dinner. Wash the dishes. Vacuum the floor. Clean the bathroom. Do the grocery shopping.

If you help with the household chores now, help a little more. That doesn't mean to take over entirely. Unless the doctor advises against it, Mom needs some exercise. Besides, the whole idea is to be working as a team, not as master and slave. (Of course, doing more than your share can be a good thing.)

Another part of your goal is to make sure that Mom realizes you are there, and always will be, standing by her side, supporting her, and, if need be, protecting her. Just remember that there is often a delicate line between being a partner and interfering (or even being a pest).

9

Is It Time?

*Y*ou've been through nine months. It's possible that neither of you knew she was pregnant for the first couple of months. That could have been followed by two or three months during which Mom's body went through some obvious changes. The two most common are mood shifts and morning sickness. Most of the second trimester was probably rather uneventful.

The last three months really make it clear that you are about to have a baby. The child grows inside, while Mom grows outside (so to speak). Especially in the last month, she is likely to become increasingly uncomfortable. Most women wait anxiously for "the time" to come, at least in part because they can hardly wait to have it all over.

Both of you are liable to be anxious for another reason. How will you know when "the time" actually comes?

Even mothers who have given birth to several children

can easily misinterpret the symptoms and go rushing to the hospital, only to find that it's a false alarm. If this happens, don't be embarrassed—and never tease Mom about it! It's not always easy to tell. Contractions and other signs can lead anyone, even the doctor, into believing that the birth is imminent.

At the other end, there are times when there are no symptoms, and suddenly Mom is in late labor. (There have been a few extremely rare cases when the only "symptom" was the sudden appearance of a baby at her feet.)

Emily had been to her regular doctor's appointment late on a Tuesday morning. She went in with anticipation. That day was the date predicted nine months before. Although she knew that very few women actually deliver on their due date, it was a disappointment when the doctor told her that it would be at least another week.

Just a matter of hours later, she felt some light pangs. By four in the afternoon, they'd become strong enough for her to lie down on the couch. At five, her husband had the watch out and was timing them. By six, he placed a call to the doctor. There was obviously *something* going on, but the indicators were far from certain.

A contraction (which is what they turned out to be) might last a few seconds, or as long as a minute. The time between was sometimes twenty or thirty seconds, and sometimes more than a half hour. On top of all this, the doctor had done a complete exam, including pelvic, just that morning. There was no blood or other fluid. No headache or dizziness. No symptoms of potential trouble at all, other than the sporadic contractions.

The doctor recommended that they keep close tabs on it for another couple of hours and call him back. By ten that night, it had been more of the same all along. The contractions *seemed* to be getting closer together, but there was still no real pattern. The doctor wasn't convinced that labor had started, but knew that it would be best to have Emily checked.

Through all of this, Emily had that elusive maternal instinct that she was definitely in labor. When they arrived at the hospital, the doctor had already called Admitting. Everything was ready. A nurse was waiting to perform an exam. "You're already six centimeters," she told Emily. She smiled at Emily, patted her on the shoulder, and said, "Yes, this is the real thing. I'll go call the doctor."

If a highly skilled doctor can't tell from the symptoms, how can you?

Be Prepared

The truth is, there is no accurate way to predict the exact day or time. All you can do is make sure that you're ready well ahead of time. Much of this was covered in Chapter Four.

As the due date approaches, and before, have the doctor paid, the hospital paid, hospital preregistration complete, bags ready to be packed, the house clean, the baby's room ready, basic supplies ready, meals prepared for a few days, the gas tank full . . .

Make three copies of the phone numbers and names for the doctor and hospital. One copy stays by the phone. You should carry one with you, and so should Mom. (She could go into labor while away from home.) Also on that list should be the phone number of at least one close friend or relative who has volunteered to help in an emergency. (What if you're not home when it comes time for Mom to get to the hospital? What if your car won't start?)

You should know at least two separate ways to get to the hospital. If one route is closed or impeded by repairs or an accident, you have an alternate. It's not a bad idea to actually drive the routes a few times. Get used to where the traffic lights are. Find out to within a few minutes how long it takes to make the drive.

At the hospital, locate the entrances. Often the main entrance is closed late at night. You may have to use the Emergency entrance or some other door. Depending on the hospital, there may be separate parking lots. Find out well before Mom goes into labor.

Your goal is to take part in the birth. If your poor planning means that you get to the hospital late, or can't find the entrance, or can't find a place to park, you might miss out.

Many hospitals offer a free car seat to new parents. If yours doesn't, get one of your own (or, rather, one for each child). This is a critical item to have after the baby's birth. It's not only foolish to hold the baby in the car, in many states it's illegal, and for good reason. Should you have an accident, there is no way to hold on to or protect the infant.

As mentioned in Chapter Four, the best place for the car seat is in the center of the car's backseat, and with the baby facing the rear of the car. This position provides maximum safety.

Signs and Symptoms

After the first exam, the doctor will calculate a delivery date. During the pregnancy, exams and symptoms may cause this anticipated date to change. This date isn't a goal or target, it's merely a rough guide. Pregnancy and birthing is not a precision manufacturing process. Even if it were possible to spot the exact second of conception, it takes *approximately* thirty-eight weeks from that point for full fetal development and birth. *Approximately* can mean almost anything. The delivery might come early, or might come late.

It's possible that there will be few symptoms to even let you know it's about to happen. It's even more possible that the symptoms and indicators that have you rushing to the hospital are caused by something else. Consequently, what follows can provide only some guidelines, and those only for the "classic" pregnancy.

A week to a month before delivery, Mom will experience lightening. She'll be able to breathe more easily, and may even feel lighter, because the baby has lowered in the uterus, with its head settled into the pelvis and ready for birth. (Note that a woman who has had children before may not experience lightening until labor has started.)

Backaches also get worse. The cause is again the change in position of the baby, and also the ever-increasing weight. With the latter comes a greater change in the center of balance, which puts unusual strains on the muscles of her lower back. All this has been going on in the last weeks, but as the birth itself approaches, the backache might become very painful.

Fairly often, Mom will lose a pound or two in the week before going into labor. Her hormones have changed again to prepare her for birthing. This brings on an increased fluid loss, causing an even greater and more frequent need to urinate.

Nature works its miracle again as labor approaches. In the last day before the birth, many women not only have the need to urinate often but will have diarrhea as well. It's almost as though her body knows that it needs to do an internal cleaning—that it needs to empty the bladder and the bowel.

Vomiting is also possible. It's likely that the causes include changes in the hormones and changes in the pressures caused by the baby. Assuming she has been getting rid of fluids and even solids (urination and diarrhea), her body is undergoing other changes as well.

You or she may notice an increase in fluids from the vagina. One of these is often called *bloody show*, sometimes simply called *show*. It's a good indicator that Mom is in labor, or is about to be. All this time, the cervix has been sealed shut with a mucus plug. It keeps the uterus as a sterile environment. Although this plug may come loose and discharge days before the birth, often it doesn't until just a matter of hours before the baby is born. This discharge will usually have a mucuslike appearance, sometimes with chunks of solid matter, and will be lightly tinged with blood. Don't be concerned if you miss the "show," but *do* be concerned if the discharge is bright red and very bloody.

The amniotic sac may or may not burst. This "bursting of the waters" happens at the beginning of labor or before in only about 10 percent of all pregnancies. It may occur days ahead of the birthing. The water is more likely to break during labor. It's possible that the doctor will have to manually rupture the sac. More rarely, the baby is born with the sac still intact.

If the sac breaks before or during labor, the flow can be anything from a slow and steady trickle to a sudden gush. Whenever it happens, the doctor needs to be notified. It means that the baby is no longer protected as well. There is a risk of infection, especially if more than twenty-four hours pass.

Another risk is *cord prolapse*. If the waters have broken, the mucus plug has been released and the cervix is opening, it's possible that the umbilical cord will come out. If it does, and if the baby presses against it, all the nutrients, including oxygen, can be cut off. This is an emergency situation! It could easily require an ambulance. (For more on this, see Chapter Eleven.)

Any vaginal discharge, including the amniotic fluid, should be fairly clear. It should be odorless or have a slightly sweet scent. If it has a bad smell, or is bright red, medical help is needed immediately. Also be aware, however, that in the last weeks of pregnancy it's not unusual for the woman to leak urine. If there is any doubt which fluid is coming out, contact the doctor and have it checked.

All women experience *Braxton Hicks contractions*, although with some women these are so light that they barely feel them. These actually began back in the third month. They tend to become more noticeable, and closer together, as delivery is near. They are uterine contractions, usually painless. At times they may be strong enough that the mother mistakes them for being the true contractions of birthing.

In most cases the mother won't confuse the Braxton Hicks contractions for the real thing, at least not once the true contractions have started. Contractions that happen five times in an hour may indicate a premature birth. Near full term, this can still be an indicator but is not as critical as with a preterm birth.

True contractions tend to be regular and strong. Many women report that the contractions feel like waves. The contraction builds to a crest, then declines. Usually, at the beginning of labor they last about fifteen seconds and take place perhaps a half hour apart. As labor proceeds, the contractions last longer and come closer together. The classic advice is that when the contractions are five minutes apart, it's time to get to the hospital.

Before you count on this absolutely, remember Emily's story from earlier in this chapter. Irregular contractions, especially those that change when the mother changes her activity (for example, if she gets up and walks), are often a sign of false labor. In Emily's case, after the first call to the doctor, they were told to wait. If they had waited until the contractions were regular and five minutes apart, the baby would have been born at home. Also be aware that although labor usually lasts about twelve to eighteen hours, it can go much faster, or much slower.

Inside, the cervix will begin to soften and dilate. The doctor or nurse will check this. (Do not try to check it at home!) Labor is "official" when the cervix has dilated to four centimeters. It is fully open at ten centimeters.

As the labor progresses, the contractions last longer, come closer together, and are more intense. They also become more painful. Although the worst of it is toward the end, just before the birth, even the contractions in the early part of labor can be painful. There are no outward signs, but Mom will almost certainly know.

The baby will probably have stopped moving around fairly early in the labor. This doesn't mean that anything is wrong or that the baby is dying. It's perfectly normal. It also stresses the importance of Mom having steady and regular medical exams. An unborn that stops moving can indicate a serious problem.

In all, your best indicator is Mom herself. She could mistake what she is feeling and cause a false alarm. It's even possible that she is so anxious to have the baby that she'll take the mildest twinge to be the first contractions of labor.

When in doubt, and especially when *not* in doubt, call the doctor. Not only can the doctor better interpret the symptoms (usually), he can phone ahead to the hospital for you. Then you can concentrate on taking care of Mom and getting there. By the time you arrive, they'll be ready.

The doctor has probably already told Mom to not take a tub bath, but rather a shower. This becomes even more critical now. A bath can allow water to get into the vagina, where it can cause a variety of problems. This is far less likely with a shower. In addition, a nice, hot shower can cause a "false labor" to go away. (It will have no similar effect if the labor is real.) If nothing else, that shower will get Mom clean and ready. If this is the real thing, Mom could easily be in labor for twenty-four hours, much of which is hard, sweaty, messy work. It's best to begin it clean. (Don't forget your own shower!)

The "Nesting Instinct"

Typically one or two days before labor begins, Mom will show a burst of energy. She'll seem to have an almost insatiable urge to clean and straighten the house, called the nesting instinct. (Don't be too surprised if you feel it, too.)

It sounds almost funny in childbirth classes—like some little bird building a nest. Essentially that's exactly what it is. Somehow nature has instilled an automatic response on the part of the mother (and sometimes the father) to prepare the nest for the young.

It can be quite disconcerting to the anxious father.

Marianne's labor pains were minutes apart. As she showered before heading for the hospital, her husband, John, hauled the suitcases and other needed items to the car, and began shutting down the house. He came back inside to find his wife vacuuming the carpet.

"Get ready to go," he suggested.

"I'm almost ready. Where is the brown suitcase?"

"It's already in the car."

"Bring it in. I need it."

She headed for the bedroom for the last-minute packing, and he headed for the car. When he came back in with the requested suitcase, Marianne was nowhere to be found. A search revealed that she was in what would be the baby's room, folding blankets.

He finally got her down the hall, out the door, and buckled into the car, then ran back into the house to get the suitcase. On his way to the door, he noticed that the lights were on in the kitchen. There was Marianne, washing dishes.

"Just these last few," she told him.

It's not uncommon for the entire day to go like that. Even before the mother feels inside that the time has come, something else tells her to get the house ready. She can run Dad ragged at such a time. Her energy seems like a bottomless well. Trying to get her to move in what seems to be a more needed direction can be frustrating.

The father might even begin to wonder if she actually realizes just how important the birth is. She's a matter of hours from giving birth, and all she can think about is cleaning the toilet or sweeping the floor.

Resist the temptation to drag her from the house. Certainly don't expect your efforts to get her to slow down to be effective. They won't help. That so-called nesting instinct can be a powerful force.

Checking in—and What Happens Next

Exactly what happens depends a lot on how well you've prepared. Of course, since you've read this far, you're probably well prepared!

If you are, the hospital will not only know that you're on the way, all the details will be taken care of. In such a case, checking in is little more than a matter of walking in and saying, "Here we are."

On the other hand, if you've been sitting back and doing nothing all those months, you'll be walking into the hospital as strangers. There are a lot of details to be taken care of before you can gain admission. There will be paperwork to fill out, releases to sign, and checks to write.

It's possible—even probable—that the hospital will go ahead and take Mom up to the labor and delivery room if the birth is obviously imminent or if there is an emergency. Meanwhile, Dad is going to be stuck in Admissions trying to take care of all the red tape. By the time all this is done, it might be too late.

Money makes the world go round. It also makes the hospital go round. In many cases, before you (or in this case, your wife) can be admitted to the hospital, you have to prove that you can pay the bill. Quite often this means that you pay it up front, even if you have health insurance. (The time to pay it off in installments is before, not after. Going to the hospital isn't like buying a car or a house.)

You'll also have to sign various release forms. At least one will release the hospital from liability. Another will release the doctor(s) from the same thing. Still another is a permission form giving the doctor and hospital the right to do what they think is best, up to and including surgical procedures for both mother and baby, and any medications for either.

Mom, and hopefully you, will be taken to the labor room. In many hospitals today, the same room serves as the delivery and recovery room as well. It's possible but fairly unlikely that the doctor will be there. It is more likely that a nurse will examine Mom. The purpose is to determine her overall condition, and also to learn if she is really in labor or if this is a false alarm.

The nurse will perform a vaginal exam to check the cervix and the baby's position. It used to be common practice to give the mother an enema to clear the bowel. Today this is rare and is almost never standard procedure. Also in the past it was common for the entire pubic area to be shaved. These days if she is shaved at all, it will be only across the perineum, and even this minor shaving is being phased out.

You may or may not be present for this. Even if you are, if the nurse determines that the labor is real, you will be given a hospital gown and possibly paper shoe covers and a cap as well. It's important to keep the area sterile. After this, the nurse will probably leave to notify the doctor as to Mom's condition. (After the exam, the nurse's training can often predict the actual time of delivery with amazing accuracy.)

Especially with a first child, labor tends to be long. It's not at all uncommon to be in the labor room for twelve hours or more (depending on how long you wait before going in). Most of this time the two of you will be alone. There's not much anyone can do (from a medical standpoint) other than to sit back and wait.

Various monitors may be used. One common method is to have a belt strapped across Mom's tummy. A sensor sends signals to a monitoring device to measure the number, timing, and intensity of the contractions. Often there will be a printout from the machine. It may also be connected to a remote monitor.

Unless there are complications, and assuming that proper care has been given to Mom throughout the pregnancy, the doctor probably won't show up until nearly the last minute. You might not like this idea, but there is no reason for him to be sitting there for hours while dilation and effacement become complete.

It's unlikely that the obstetric nurse will be with you constantly, either. Once again, there's really no need.

Eating and Drinking

There are varying opinions on whether Mom should have anything to eat or drink when she knows she is in labor. At one time doctors recommended that she eat or drink nothing at all, other than water. That was at a time when general anesthesia was also more common. This can upset the stomach and cause vomiting, which can cause other troubles. Today most doctors search for a careful balance.

It's well known that the digestive system slows during labor and comes to a complete stop late in the game. This means that a heavy meal, or a meal of hard-to-digest foods, should be avoided. Generally also to be avoided are acidic products, such as coffee, citrus juices, etc. Doctors sometimes recommend a light meal. Cottage cheese, pasta, broth, and yogurt are examples.

It can become a careful balance. Labor can last for twenty-four hours and longer. If Mom goes into labor just before dinner, her last meal was lunch or an afternoon snack. This is not the time for her to be fasting. She needs her strength and energy.

The basic rule of thumb is the same as always—ask the doctor!

During labor it's rare for the mother to be offered anything other than ice chips and perhaps some low-acid juice. More likely is that an IV will be attached, through which she will be given fluids and glucose. Especially in a long labor, there is the potential danger of her becoming dehydrated, and also of running out of energy. The IV also gives the medical staff an easy way to administer any needed medications.

What Can You Do?

The first key is to be prepared. Take care of as many details as possible before it becomes necessary to deal with them. This will reduce stress and make everything move more smoothly. There will be enough to do just dealing with the labor, birth, and the new baby.

Being prepared will also help you to remain calm. This is important for you, and is even more important for Mom. All the support you've provided during the pregnancy climaxes in the birthing. You become her source of strength.

There are no exact answers. Each pregnancy, and each birthing, is different. Probably the best guideline is "Go with the flow." If Mom seems to want her back rubbed, rub it. If she yells for you to stop, then stop.

You might find that even things the two of you have practiced just don't work in reality. For example, during the pregnancy there might have been a focal object used—something for Mom to concentrate on during labor. As the contractions grow in intensity, she may lose all interest in this, and may demand that you "shut off that stupid music!"

This is okay, too.

Your presence alone means more than you might realize. Even if she yells insults at you, a purpose is being served. You become a focal point of sorts. She can focus on you, outside herself, which really does help.

Remember that childbirth hurts. Your loved one is going to be in pain for a number of hours. Especially toward the end, that pain can be severe. Your support and words of encouragement and love can make a considerable difference. You're likely to read or hear a lot about bonding with the baby. What is often forgotten, or ignored, is the bonding between the mother and the father.

Birthing can do that. It begins months before, and continues after the birth. The experience of being there can be one of the most incredible events in your life—and in your *lives,* as a couple.

10

Labor and Birth

*T*he last chapter concentrated on recognizing when Mom goes into labor, driving to the hospital, and getting ready for what is to come. This chapter assumes that labor has been determined, and that you are now at the hospital (or other birthing facility or arrangement).

At this point the mucus plug has come out, although it's possible that both of you missed it. It's possible, but fairly unlikely, that the waters have broken. What is almost certain is that from the beginning, Mom will become increasingly uncomfortable. Even those first contractions can hurt. The later ones certainly will. In addition, she could have a backache, cramps, and muscle spasms. She could become nauseated and may vomit.

On the other hand, once she has checked into the hospital and labor has been confirmed, she *could* become quite relaxed. You've been waiting for this moment for months.

She has been waiting, too, but more so. Especially during that last month, many women just want it all over.

Over the next hours, the two of you have the opportunity to share in something very special. This isn't just her time, it's *your* time, too. Together, the two of you conceived a child. Together, you've gone through the pregnancy. You're about to go through the birthing together.

It's true that Mom has been doing most of the "work," and is about to do more. All you can do is imagine what it's like to be pregnant and to give birth. Being male, you'll never have this experience directly. That doesn't mean you're totally outside.

Mom needs you through these hours!

On the average, labor rarely lasts less than two hours or more than twenty-four hours, with labor in a first pregnancy tending to be longer. Expect it to go from being uncomfortable to painful and beyond. Most women can handle early labor without too much difficulty. In the middle stages the contractions get stronger and come more often.

Toward the end, there is no doubt that the ordeal is something you'd avoid. Even with painkillers, her body is going through a lot. Five minutes after, she's likely to be sweeter and nicer than you've ever known her to be. Despite her screams and cussing during transition and the birth, just minutes later she could be saying, "That wasn't much. I bet our baby would like a baby sister."

The birth itself is messy. Be ready for it. The amniotic sac bursts most often late in labor, flooding the labor table. It's possible that Mom will urinate or empty what remains in her bowels. Beyond that, even in a "clean" birth there will be blood. And your wife will be in pain.

At a minimum, with a vaginal birth the baby will come out with a misshapen head and is unlikely to have that healthy glow and color to the skin (although this usually comes very quickly). The child could be coated with white, messy caul or vernix. The blood covering the child is the mother's (and is not necessarily a sign of danger).

Many people think that the baby is somewhat (or entirely) repulsive when it first emerges. At this point it's gooey and gray and misshapen and covered with blood. Bill Cosby described it quite well. According to him, at the birth of his child he turned to his wife and said, "You've just had . . . a lizard."

Don't be surprised if you find a bit of panic swelling up inside. You might worry that you have a grossly deformed baby. You might even look at it and wonder if it's even alive. Such thoughts are quite common in first-timers.

Despite this, if you're prepared, you can enjoy, and participate in, the wonder of it all.

Stages of Labor

There are a number of ways to define labor. The most common is to divide it into stages. Stage one is the labor up to the birth. Stage two is the birth itself. Stage three is usually called the afterbirth, which is delivery of the placenta. Sometimes each stage is further subdivided, especially the first stage. This stage is usually subdivided as early labor, middle labor, and transition.

In childbirth class, or in other books you read, other terms may be used. Don't let yourself be confused. However it is defined, and whatever terms are used, it's the same thing. It's generally a steady, progressive process with many variables.

Labor begins with uterine contractions and release of the mucus plug over the cervix. As labor progresses, the contractions come closer together and get stronger. The cervix softens and opens. After some hours, the baby moves down the birth canal and is delivered.

Once the baby has been born, the placenta has to be removed. This often happens in much the same manner as birthing the baby—that is, uterine contractions expel the placenta. The doctor may need to intervene. The baby is examined. So is the placenta. If all has gone well, you have become parents and will be home in a day or two.

Early Labor

Some define early labor as starting with the very first contractions. The problem with this is that Mom may experience contractions for many days before the actual birth. It's not unusual for contractions to begin, then stop for days or longer, begin again, stop again.

This leads others to define early labor as being when contractions begin, remain steady, and come closer and closer. Although this is usually fairly reliable, it's possible (although rare) that there will be no real pattern. She might have two contractions within a few minutes, then nothing for another ten minutes.

The most common medical definition of early labor relies on the opening (dilation) of the cervix, with early labor being the dilation from closed to four centimeters. This is about the same as two fingers (but do NOT try to check this yourself!). Much of the time, the nurse or doctor won't declare that labor has "officially" begun until the cervix has dilated to four centimeters.

At this point contractions are usually lasting between thirty and sixty seconds and are about five minutes apart. If you haven't already called the doctor, that should be done now. He can advise you, and can also call ahead to the hospital.

Bloody show, often simply called "the show," will happen, if it hasn't already. This is the release of the mucus plug that has kept the cervix sealed all these months. The term describes a vaginal discharge that has a mucuslike appearance that is probably tinged lightly with blood. You may or may not see anything solid. Far more important is the color. A slight bloodiness is okay and even to be expected. There should *not* be a lot of blood. This is the sign of hemorrhage, which is a full medical emergency.

There may or may not be fluid from the amniotic sac. In 85 percent of pregnancies, the sac doesn't break until much later. If the amniotic sac does break, the flow may be a steady trickle or a sudden gush. The fluid should be clear and odorless, but might have a slightly sweet smell. If it's red (colored with blood) or has a bad odor, don't wait any longer. Call the doctor and get to the hospital.

Mom might experience a backache. Much of the time this is normal and not of any concern (other than Mom's comfort). The pain shouldn't be severe, however. If it is, the cause could be that the baby is in such a position that it is applying pressure. This could be an indication that a vaginal birthing may be difficult or impossible. Assuming Mom has been attending the doctor's appointments, you'll probably know by now if the backache is a problem, or merely the chance for you to pamper her a bit more with a back rub.

She might feel nauseated, to the point of vomiting. If she hasn't already had diarrhea in the last couple of days, this could come at the onset of labor. As previously stated, it's as though nature is trying to clean and empty her system for the ordeal of giving birth.

Her digestive system has slowed all through pregnancy. During labor it will slow even further and eventually come to a stop. This, the need to empty the bowel and bladder, and the nausea she could experience mean that any meals she takes even very early in labor should be extremely light. During labor in the hospital, about all she'll be offered will be chips of ice, with these meant mostly to help keep her mouth and throat moist. In other words, this isn't the time to have dinner.

Once again the doctor can advise you. This requires a balance. If Mom eats, she could have increased problems with urination, bowel movements, and vomiting. If she doesn't eat, and considering that it could be twenty-four hours and more before delivery, plus some hours for recovery . . . well, this isn't the time for fasting, either.

Mid First Stage

The middle of labor is usually defined as the period during which the cervix dilates from four centimeters to eight. At the beginning, the examining nurse will feel an opening about two fingers wide, and at the end all four fingers could be inserted into the cervical opening.

Her contractions become stronger. Each lasts between forty-five and ninety seconds and will be approximately three minutes apart. Even if the fetal presentation is ideal, it's likely that Mom will have backaches and leg pains. With this come two tricky situations for you.

First, it's not unusual for Mom to sleep through much of the early and middle parts of labor. Some of the contractions will be strong enough to wake her. If a monitor is attached to record the contractions, which is fairly common, you will notice a number of contractions showing on the readout, and Mom sleeping blissfully through them. If you notice that she has gone to sleep, let her rest.

It's easy for the first-time father to panic. (One father buzzed the attending nurse, afraid that his wife had passed into a coma and was dying.) Why can't she remain conscious? This can be especially puzzling if you've had it drilled into you how painful labor and birthing are. By all means, keep your eye on Mom, and on the monitor. It's not difficult to tell the difference between someone who is sleeping and someone who is in trouble.

Second, aches and pains can often be helped by massage. Many childbirth classes recommend that you bring special "tools" along for this, such as wooden rollers. Hopefully at least some basic massage techniques have become familiar due to practicing them during the pregnancy. You should be all set to take care of this.

Some women love being touched and rubbed right through the birth. Others will take a swing at you if you so much as try to hold their hand. Still others will make things more confusing by constantly changing. This is more common in the final phase (transition), but can begin anytime during labor.

This same thing can make it difficult for you to coach and help with the breathing exercises. It's also why it is so important to practice ahead of time. Mom isn't likely to be interested in trying something new and unfamiliar at this particular time.

A large part of your job is to provide reassurance. If this began during the pregnancy (or ideally, before that), your presence and the occasional "You're doing great, honey" can help take the edge off. On the other hand, be prepared for her to snap at you about how you haven't the slightest idea of what she is going through, and to call you names.

Early in labor, she'll probably handle the contractions just fine. There is also a rest period between them. During mid labor (sometimes called "active labor," and for good reason), the contractions come closer together and with greater strength. Other than the breathing and relaxing techniques you learned in childbirth class—and hopefully practiced at home—one of the best things you can do is to encourage Mom to handle each contraction, one at a time. This helps her to focus on the moment, rather than to fret about what is to come.

It also helps if she concentrates on only the first half of the contraction. Remember that the contractions swell like a wave, then peak, then subside. Once the contraction peaks, "it's all downhill." Assuming that a monitor is attached, you can help by watching it. That way you can let Mom know when the contraction has peaked.

This simple technique can help Mom through active labor, transition, and the birth itself. It will also help her work *with* the contractions instead of fighting them. In turn, this will make the process go faster while giving Mom an effective way to deal with the pain.

Transition

During the final phase, called transition, the cervix opens completely to ten centimeters. This phase rarely lasts more than an hour. Knowing this can help both of you get through it. Mom is going to be in pain. It's good to know that the pain is not only natural and normal, it's a sign that in a short time it will all be over—and you will be parents.

Contractions have become severe and painful. Even if Mom entered into labor determined to use no drugs, she may ask for something now. It's common for the medical staff to offer the mother a painkiller—rather, a pain-softener—even if she doesn't ask. If so, it does not mean she has failed in any way. Also, many times the medication to lessen the pain can help Mom to not fight the contractions. (It's natural for anyone to fight against pain.)

The most common medication is Demerol, which is a synthetic morphine. The purpose is to alleviate the pain while keeping the amount of drugs to a bare minimum. Demerol is one of the safest, although it, like any other drug, can cause complications.

Although reducing the pain can help Mom work with the contractions, sometimes it relaxes the woman too much. The contractions aren't as strong, which can lead to a longer labor time. In some cases this has caused enough exhaustion in the mother that a normal vaginal birth was impossible. Some claim that the use of drugs such as Demerol is directly related to the increased number of C-sections.

Another fairly common method of pain control is *epi-*

dural anesthesia. For this, a small needle is inserted into the spine, with drops of anesthetic put in. This numbs the lower body. Usually it is given only during active labor and stopped before transition. This relieves pain while still allowing Mom to push. The advantage is that since it is directed medication, less is needed, and less gets to baby. One disadvantage is that it numbs the legs, which forces Mom to stay in bed. She can't walk to help speed the labor. This and the general numbing effect can force a forceps delivery. In addition, some women become nauseated from the drug and may vomit.

With or without medication, the contractions during transition are often "stacked." They last sixty to ninety seconds, and come about a minute apart. As stated previously, each contraction comes as a wave, building to a peak and then subsiding. During transition, as one contraction is subsiding, the next may be building. They come one after another (hence the term "stacking"), with little or no rest between.

With the contractions come cramps, hot and cold flashes, heavy perspiration, and possible nausea. It's a good idea to have a towel on hand for cleanup, just in case.

It's very common for Mom to feel the desire to push. The nurse or doctor will warn her against it. She shouldn't push until the cervix is fully dilated. You won't know when this is, so it is better to let the medical staff handle the situation. They'll know when she should hold back and when she should push.

In the last section you were warned that Mom is likely to be highly emotional. If she wasn't in the second phase, she almost certainly will be now. The doctor and nurse are used to this, and even expect it. You should, too. Don't take anything she says personally. This is not a matter of her releasing hidden hostilities or anger. She is merely lashing out at the pain. Those around her are handy focal points for this. Chances are pretty good that after the baby is born, Mom won't remember much, or anything, of what she said. Neither should you.

She often doesn't want to be touched. Things that helped earlier may hurt now, or may at least be irritating. It could be that the only contact she wants is to have you give her ice chips. There is no way to know or to predict exactly what will happen, what she'll want, or how you can help. Remain aware, and just do the best you can.

Second Stage—the Birth

Once the cervix is fully open, the baby's head passes through and into the birth canal. Fortunately, the vagina is remarkably flexible. Normally it remains closed. It can expand to accept the penis—roughly about one inch in diameter. During birth it expands even farther to allow passage of the baby. After the birth, the vagina returns to normal (or nearly so).

This is amazing, but it's also painful. It doesn't take much imagination to understand. Even a small baby is a fairly large object to have pass through the birth canal. One comedian described it as having a bowel movement that is trying to pass a watermelon.

Mom's urge to push increases. The contractions come further apart. The doctor will be monitoring the progress and will direct her when to push and when to hold back. On the average, she will be directed to push three times during each contraction, and to relax as completely as possible between.

Your job as "coach" is to encourage her to push (at the doctor's direction) during the contractions and to relax between. Help her through the breathing and relaxing techniques you have practiced. Watch her face. This will give you clues as to whether she is relaxed.

The length of time it takes for the baby to make that short journey varies. It could be a matter of minutes, or could be much longer. If it takes too long, the doctor may have to intervene. Typical is to administer a drug such as oxytocin. This helps to make the contractions stronger.

You may read or hear that one way to stimulate natural production of oxytocin is to rub her nipples. Although a valid technique, this may not be welcome. It can be embarrassing for her. It can also be painful or irritating.

The doctor may decide that forceps are needed to assist in the delivery. In a comedy routine, Bill Cosby told of how he screamed at the doctor, "Get the salad spoons!" This is a fair description. There are different kinds of forceps, but all serve the same basic function. They are used to grasp the baby's head so it can be pulled down the birth canal.

In a more serious case, the baby has trouble getting through the cervix. Again oxytocin or some other drug might be used. The doctor will be watching Mom carefully. Contractions alone are rarely enough to deliver the baby. This is why Mom is directed to push. She will be told to work with the contractions, and relax between. Both are important. Labor is called labor for good reason. It's hard work! And painful. If Mom reaches the point of exhaustion before the baby has been delivered vaginally, forceps or C-section may be the only options left.

There isn't much you can do about this. The best help you can provide is reassurance and a positive attitude.

Assuming all goes well, eventually the top of the baby's head will appear. It's called crowning (because the crown of the baby's head shows). Many women describe the sensation as being something similar to an "Indian burn."

At this point the doctor will become more cautious again. If Mom pushes too hard, or pushes at the wrong time, the tissues at the opening of the vagina and of the perineum might tear. Now more than ever it is important that Mom work with the contractions, one at a time.

Finally the head emerges. Many times the shoulders also

have to be coaxed. After this, the rest of the birth tends to be quick and sudden.

Your place through most of this is by Mom's side. The doctor or nurse will probably announce that the baby is crowning. This is more for Mom's benefit than yours. She needs that encouragement. Pick up on it. "You're almost there!"

It's also a signal to you. Your baby is very nearly born at this point. This is something you may want to see. Hopefully you'll also be right there as the delivery is completed. Be prepared for the mess. There will be blood and other fluids. The baby will also be covered. Its head will have an odd shape due to passage through the pelvis and birth canal. It's not at all unusual for the baby to be discolored in some way.

Think back to the story at the beginning of this book. There a new father hadn't been told what to expect and went into a total panic thinking that he'd just become the father of a deformed monster. If he'd waited just a little while, the nurse would have had time to clean the baby. The baby would have had time to begin breathing and bring a more normal coloring to the skin.

Also be aware that Mom might need you in those last few minutes. It could be more important that you be at her side, helping to support her, than it is to be down with the doctor ready to catch the baby. This varies, and again there is no way to predict it. Being right there when your baby is delivered is important. So is being at Mom's side.

The doctor will clear the fluid and mucus from the breathing passages. In a matter of moments the baby will take its first breaths, and will object to being yanked from its warm and safe environment of the womb by crying vigorously.

Attached to the baby and running up inside the mother between her legs is the umbilical cord. It will be about a half inch in diameter and look something like a colorful rope. Pink and gray and red and blue. This will remain attached for a few minutes until all the blood completes its transition into the baby's body and the cord stops pulsing. It doesn't hurt to leave the cord intact too long (within reason, of course) and can be a detriment if it's cut too soon.

The doctor will clamp off the umbilical in two places somewhere between an inch and about four inches from the baby's body. Quite often it will be double-clamped on the baby's side, and then single-clamped on the placental side. The cut goes between the two clamps.

Later the umbilical will be tied and/or clamped close to the baby's body. The little stub will slowly dry up and within a week or so will fall off.

The doctor will hand the baby to the nurse and turn back to the mother. There will be a somewhat lengthy process of delivering the afterbirth, checking the same, then cleaning and patching up any tears or surgical cuts. Much of this goes unnoticed by both the father and mother.

Meanwhile the nurse will clean up the baby and will be giving it at least two Apgar scores—at one minute and again at five minutes. The Apgar tests are named after Dr. Virginia Apgar of Columbia University. The score is zero through ten, with ten being perfect. The five areas involve heart rate, respiration, muscle tone, response to stimulation, and skin color. A score of zero is the worst (e.g., doesn't respond), with two being the best. A score of seven or higher is considered to be normal—although a score of zero in any category is cause for concern.

Third Stage—Afterbirth

Once the baby has been delivered, still inside the uterus is the placenta. It has taken care of the baby all those months. Now it must be removed. This process can take between five minutes and (rarely) an hour.

The mother often doesn't realize that it is happening.

Uterine contractions continue. The placenta is delivered much as the baby was, but Mom has reached the point of relief, elation, and exhaustion. Unless there are complications, the doctor will be able to remove the placenta, stitch the episiotomy or any tearing, and clean her up, without Mom noticing much at all.

The placenta is usually placed in a pan. It is then examined carefully to be sure that none of it remains in the uterus. If it does, the mother could hemorrhage or have other problems. The doctor may have to reach up through the already expanded vaginal canal and cervix to remove any pieces. If this isn't possible, surgery similar to a C-section may become necessary.

In the majority of cases, the afterbirth goes smoothly.

The New Baby

Within about five minutes the baby will start looking like a little human being. Assuming a vaginal birth, the head will almost certainly still be misshapen. This will remain for several weeks. Eventually it will go away, so don't worry about it.

For a while the baby's eyesight is rather poor. His or her whole world is a blur. His eyes are also quite sensitive to light. (Some have even suggested that birthing should take place in a darkened room to help make baby's first minutes more pleasant and less of a shock.)

Babies have a natural tendency to look at faces. Put a toy in front of the baby and he will probably ignore it. Put a face in front of him and he might give you his first smile.

Nature has done a wonderful thing. The baby's range of sight extends to only about twelve inches, and he has that natural fondness for looking at faces. It just happens that when the baby is put to the mother's breast for its first feeding, he is right in front of a face and at just the right distance.

More and more experts are suggesting that the mother should, if at all possible, breast-feed the baby right on the delivery table. Many say that this should take place even while the umbilical is still attached. Breast-feeding stimulates oxytocin. This helps deliver the placenta, and also serves to help reduce bleeding.

It also makes the baby's first experience with the outside more pleasant. Think about what the baby is going through. He has been comfortably lolling around in the mother's womb—warm and pleasant and comfortable. Then all of a sudden his head and body are squeezed and crushed as they pass between the pelvic bones and down through the small birth canal. After being banged around for several hours, he pops out into a room that is probably twenty degrees or so colder than anything he has ever experienced.

On the mother's stomach, or at her breast, he feels the warmth. Many say that he can sense the mother's familiar heartbeat, just as he did in the womb, so the world isn't a totally strange environment.

A built-in ability is that of finding the breast and sucking. It's commonly called the rooting reflex. Touch the baby's cheek and he will automatically turn his head toward what touched him and try to suck on it. The baby doesn't actually know how to breast-feed, but he'll learn *fast*! So will Mom. In the hospital, including right there on the delivery table, the nurses will help her over the awkward first times.

Depending on circumstances, the newborn may be given a quick wipe and handed to the mother, or may be taken away. This is determined by the Apgar score (as described above). If the baby has a very low score, immediate medical attention may be needed. A somewhat low score bears close watching, with the baby being checked again after five minutes or so.

Typically, even if the baby is handed to the mother right after the birth, it will be taken aside very soon. The attending nurse will clean the baby as well as check it. The cut and tied umbilical cord is checked. Antiseptic is applied to prevent infection. The baby will then be wrapped in something warm, such as a blanket. To complete the wrap, a stocking cap is often used to cover the head.

Eventually the baby is taken to the nursery for a more thorough examination, while the mother and father are taken to the room where Mom will recover to go home.

In most cases the mother recovers quickly. It used to be fairly common for the mother to spend up to a week in the hospital after the birth. A decade ago the average was two days. Today many hospitals insist that the mother go home after just one day. There are still some weeks to come for total recovery, of course.

After a suitable period, the doctor is likely to come in to at least talk to the mother, and probably to examine her. There will be a steady flow of nurses coming to the room to make sure that Mom is okay and to see to her needs.

If required, help will be given to teach her how to breast-feed the child. Films, slide strips, and a variety of other materials might be offered. More and more hospitals are taking a personal and in-depth approach. A few (too few) have even made it a point to be sure that the father feels welcome.

Most hospitals now have an open "rooming in" policy. This means that Mom can be with the baby whenever she wishes, and can also rest when she wishes. The hospital staff may make use of this time to teach her how to breast-feed and to answer any other questions either of you might have. If you've done your homework, and have attended the child-birth classes, the bulk of what remains to be learned will be the "hands-on experiences." For example, the *theory* of breast-feeding can be read in a book, but actual practice is needed. Changing a diaper on a plastic doll is quite different from changing the diaper of a real, live baby.

Make use of this time. Once you're home, you're pretty much on your own. You're now parents, with a new baby that relies on both of you. And whether Mom spends only one day or a full week in the hospital, once you're home, *she* needs you, too.

What Can You Do?

Don't worry about feeling lost. Expect it. You have an advantage if this isn't the first time you've been there with Mom through the labor and birthing. Even then, each one is likely to be different. Whether this is the first for you or the tenth, your job is the same.

Your job is to be her coach and her strength.

As the coach, your job is to help her through the things you practiced during the pregnancy, such as the breathing and relaxing techniques learned in the childbirth classes. You are the guide. At times you may need to remind her, especially during transition.

In active labor and during the birth, it's important that she relax between the contractions. This gives her some rest so that she'll have more energy when it's needed later. You may have to remind her to relax. Watch her face and listen to her breathing. You can usually tell if she is relaxing or not.

Throughout, be aware of everything. This doesn't mean you have to make constant comments. You may not make any at all. But if you are aware, you'll have a better idea of what she is going through, will notice changes, and if need be, can tell the nurse or doctor. Likewise, if the nurse or doctor tells Mom to do (or not do) a certain thing, you're there to help with this.

Your words of encouragement are an important source of strength. A simple comment like, "There's the head. I can see the head!" will go a long way toward giving Mom a second wind for those last pushes. (By that time, she will probably be exhausted.)

That encouragement should continue after the birth.

Mom is going to be exhausted, sore, and uncomfortable. Hopefully she can get some much-needed sleep (although the excitement may cut this short). If at all possible, try to be there for her when she wakes.

11

Problems

$\mathcal{I}$n some ways, no birth is without complications. It hurts, and it's messy. Days or even weeks will pass before Mom starts feeling normal again.

Fortunately, most problems that occur are easily handled by a competent professional. Life-threatening problems are extremely rare these days, and the majority of those come about because of the mother's lifestyle, such as the use of drugs or alcohol.

Up to this point we have assumed that everything will go along fairly smoothly for both of you. This chapter presents information on the most common ways that things can go wrong. As with the pregnancy and birthing in general, knowledge will go a long way toward keeping panic out of the situation.

Many of the conditions in this chapter will have been diagnosed, or at least anticipated, ahead of time. For example, if there is more than one baby, it will be discovered well before the birth. The position of the child, and even its size, will also be fairly well known. Other threats that are usually predictable are infectious or contagious diseases, an earlier C-section, physical injury that could affect the birthing, etc.

Miscarriage

No one really knows how many women suffer a miscarriage. This is because most of them happen early in the pregnancy, and sometimes before the woman even knows she is pregnant. Almost all take place before the twentieth week, with 80 percent of them occurring before twelve weeks.

The miscarriage is almost always accompanied by bleeding. If early enough, however, this may be mistaken for nothing more than a heavy period. If later, the bleeding could be more substantial. Regardless, if the woman knows she is pregnant, *any* bleeding should be reported to the doctor.

The exact cause of a miscarriage may never be known. As mentioned in Chapter Seven, about 25 percent are caused by cervical incompetence. Other times it will be brought on by something in the mother's lifestyle, such as heavy drug or alcohol use. Despite what many believe, it's fairly rare for it to be brought on by a blow to the mother's stomach. Most of the time it merely happens because the baby didn't "take."

Usually when the sperm fertilizes the egg, the egg moves down the fallopian tube into the uterus, implants itself, and begins to grow. As it grows, the cells begin to differentiate into structures that will eventually become the various organs and tissues. Sometimes this doesn't happen. The egg may not implant itself properly. Or the cell growth never differentiates.

Some advocates of abortion refer to the growing fetus as being "nothing more than a lump of protoplasm." For a normal baby, this isn't true. It takes on definite human form very quickly. But if the cells fail to differentiate, what is growing inside the mother truly is little more than that lump of protoplasm. It's not a viable human being, and the mother will miscarry.

Some take comfort in this. Others do not. Suffering a miscarriage can be emotionally devastating, to *both* the mother and father. It can bring on a deep depression that may require professional counseling. It can also bring on a fear about trying again. The woman (or the man) may lose all interest in sex.

Mostly it takes time to recover from the loss. Exactly how you handle it depends on the two of you, and on your personalities. Be there for each other, and try to be understanding.

Malpresentation

About 95 percent of the time, the baby settles into the pelvis with its head down, facing the mother's back, chin tucked and limbs folded. This is called the normal presentation. There are other positions the baby might take, however. Some of these can cause serious trouble.

During the pregnancy the doctor will be monitoring the baby's position. Depending on the kind of malpresentation, he may attempt an external version. This is a massage technique used usually in the thirty-seventh and thirty-eighth weeks. Mom is given a drug to relax the uterus. The doctor then tries to reposition baby. Even if he is successful, the baby often flips back around again anyway.

The most common malpresentation is one in which the baby faces forward instead of toward the back. If the baby is small enough, and the pelvic outlet large enough, the doctor may decide to let the birthing proceed. Most of the time he will attempt to turn the baby.

He'll often begin with massage and by having the mother get down on her hands and knees. This helps the uterus to move down and forward, which gives the baby (and the doctor) more room. If this doesn't work, he may have to reach through the vagina, either with a hand or with a forceps, to turn the baby. Should none of this work to reposition the baby, the doctor may decide that a C-section will be necessary for a safe delivery.

Sometimes the baby will be head-down and facing the back, but with the head tilted. If tilted just slightly, with the forehead coming first (brow presentation), there is a fair chance that the doctor can handle the situation and deliver the child vaginally. Tilted farther, with the face coming first, the situation is more complicated. As the baby is pushed through, the head can continue to tilt farther and farther until the baby literally becomes stuck.

A breech presentation is when the baby's feet and/or butt are down. This occurs in about 3 percent of all births, with the birth of twins being a common link. With a multiple birth, even if one baby is in the proper position, the other(s) may not be. Contrary to what you might have heard, it's often possible to complete a vaginal birthing despite a breech presentation.

One of the greatest problems is that with a breech presentation, the umbilical cord can be squeezed shut. When this happens, the blood supply is cut off and the baby begins to suffocate. The delivery must be completed in no more than eight to ten minutes, and preferably faster. For this reason many doctors automatically call for a C-section on a breech birth. (It also makes their job easier. Delivering a breech child is difficult and often risky.)

With a frank breech the baby is butt-first with the legs straight and extended over the head. Because of the position of the legs, the umbilical is given some protection. A vaginal birth is sometimes possible.

A complete breech has the baby in a lotus position. The

legs are crisscrossed. The arms are usually crossed over the face. A footling breech is when one (or both) of the legs comes out first. In both cases, a C-section is almost a certainty.

The worst malpresentation is transverse. In this, the baby is lying sideways in the uterus. It's very rare that the doctor will be able to reposition the baby. Because of this and the danger of the uterus rupturing, the doctor will almost certainly schedule a C-section and won't even attempt to start a vaginal birthing.

Placental and Umbilical Cord Problems

After conception the fertilized egg implants on the uterine wall. The placenta begins to develop and grow. In a way, it's the placenta that taps into Mom's body to provide all the nourishment and oxygen needed. This passes from the mother to the growing baby through the umbilical cord. Problems with either the placenta or the cord can be potentially life-threatening.

Abruptio placentae, also called *abruption of placenta*, occurs in fewer than 1 percent of pregnancies. The majority of these occur in women who suffer from high blood pressure, followed closely by women who have already had a previous episode of this nature. Other risk categories include black women, women over forty, and women who have had a number of children. Smoking has also been linked with this condition.

No one is completely sure why it happens, but in this condition the placenta breaks loose from the uterine wall. Even if the separation is only partial, the uterus will begin to bleed. Sometimes this will show as a vaginal discharge. Even a small bloody discharge is an indication that immediate medical attention is needed. She may also experience abdominal pains, backache, and short, rapid contractions.

Depending on the severity, the lives of both the mother

and baby might be at risk, or it might be merely a situation that requires close watching. You won't know, so don't take the chance. Sometimes what can seem minor to you is actually life-threatening. Mom could need an immediate transfusion to survive. It's also possible that the baby will have to be delivered, such as by C-section.

Vaginal bleeding can also indicate a condition called *placenta previa*. In this case the bleeding is usually painless. One of the misleading symptoms is that the bleeding sometimes stops. This and the lack of pain could cause you and the mother to think that everything is fine. This is possible, but assume it is dangerous! Any bleeding should be reported to the doctor, and especially so late in the second trimester and all through the third. The risk factors for this condition are much the same as with abruption. There also seems to be an increased risk for women who have had an abortion or C-section.

Ideally the placenta will seat and grow toward the upper part of the uterus. Lacking this, even a low-lying placenta will tend to move upward as the pregnancy goes on. The placenta can also grow near or over the cervix. If a small part of the placenta covers the cervix, the condition is considered marginal. A vaginal birth is possible. If more of the cervix is covered, the situation becomes more serious. Even a partial blockage is likely to cause hemorrhage. A total blockage makes vaginal birth impossible. In essence, the baby would have to be delivered *through* the placenta.

Keep in mind that the placenta is the main supply for the baby. It is filled with blood going to and from it. It may sound a little gross, but it's not entirely inaccurate to think of the placenta as a somewhat oversize leech attached to the uterine wall. If it breaks loose (abruption) or is ripped open from pressure against it (previa), not only is the baby's blood source threatened, Mom can bleed to death.

New techniques, such as using a sonogram, can help locate the exact location of the placenta. In the past this situation often led to the death of mother and/or child. These days, with proper care, both will be fine.

Cord prolapse is when the umbilical cord comes out ahead of the child. This is an extremely dangerous situation that requires immediate medical attention. If the cord gets pinched or squeezed shut, the baby's oxygen supply is cut off. The baby can suffocate in a matter of minutes.

If this happens in the hospital, chances are very good that the doctor will perform an emergency C-section. If you're at home, call for an ambulance immediately! While waiting, have Mom get on her hands and knees and lower her chest to the floor. This way the baby is less likely to press against the cord. *Do not* try to push the cord back inside. The most you should do, and this carefully, is to place a clean, warm, wet cloth over the cord.

Sometimes the baby becomes tangled in the cord. Once again, this is not the kind of situation you should attempt to handle. Fortunately, you probably won't have to. In the off chance that you end up having to deliver the baby on your own, there is only a small chance that the cord will be wrapped around the baby's neck or elsewhere.

The basic rule is to avoid touching the umbilical cord. If you must, such as to unwrap it from the baby, do so only with very clean hands, and then very gently. Never yank or pull. Remain calm.

C-section

With a C-section, the cost of the birthing can more than triple. (Does your insurance cover this? Or will you need to plan and save ahead?) Mom's stay at the hospital will go from a day or two to about a week. Recovery time afterward is also increased.

Any operation brings potential dangers. This particular operation, however, has relatively few risks. In other words, if the operation becomes necessary, don't panic. Most of the time it's so routine that the father is invited to attend. Usually the operation takes about an hour. (In an emergency, it will go much faster.)

In America about 25 percent of the births are C-sections. Some claim that this is far too frequent and say that too many doctors resort to performing a C-section without valid reason. Others say that this claim is false and that C-sections are never done unless needed. No doubt the debate will continue.

Sometimes there is no choice. If the baby is in a transverse (sideways) position, it's highly unlikely that a vaginal birth will be possible. The mother might have a communicable disease that would be passed to the baby if born vaginally. This doesn't eliminate the controversy.

Jennifer's child is approaching seven years old. Even now she still complains that the doctor opted for a C-section too soon. "I feel violated," she says. "He was watching the clock, not me, and he robbed me of a great experience."

Some doctors use a timetable of sorts. The idea is that after a certain amount of time, the mother will be exhausted and no longer able to push well enough to give birth vaginally. Jennifer feels that this is what happened to her.

Another controversy concerns fetal distress. Often electronic fetal monitors are used. If the indication is that the baby is in trouble, the doctor may go to a C-section. Some claim that this is done too quickly, especially since the monitor may be inaccurate, or the readings misinterpreted.

Jennifer's story reflects what many women feel. It's entirely possible that the doctor was aware of something she wasn't. Knowing that doesn't always help. There could be the sense of disappointment or even of failure. She might feel that all choices were taken out of her hands. It's true that sometimes this happens, but it's probably not as common as some claim. Most of the time there is a valid reason for the operation. There are also some who welcome it.

Beth is pregnant with her second child. Her first child was a footling breech, which forced a C-section. Now her doctor wants her to attempt VBAC (vaginal birth after C-section). She's very frightened. "With a C-section, I know what to expect," she says.

Regardless, it's a very good idea to discuss this with the doctor early in the pregnancy. You need to find out how he feels about C-section. He should have at least some idea of how many babies he has delivered, and how many C-sections he has performed. This tells you two things. One is how competent he is to perform the operation if it becomes necessary. The other is how quick he is to go this route. If the percentage is low, you know that he will try every other means first. If it's high, either he has had a large number of "at risk" patients, or *might* use the operation too soon, too often.

Often it is known ahead of time that a C-section will be needed. Other times the decision will be made in the delivery room. There are a number of reasons the operation might be needed.

A woman carrying twins (or more) is likely to need the procedure. It's fairly unusual for the babies to all be in the right position for a vaginal birth. Even if one is in a perfect position, the other may not be. Depending on how far off things are, the doctor may attempt a vaginal birthing, or may schedule the operating room for a C-section ahead of time.

Cephalopelvic disproportion (CPD) is the fancy term used to say that the baby's head is too large to get through the pelvic outlet and down the birth canal. From the very first examination the doctor has attempted to determine potential problems in this regard. He'll try to approximate the size of the opening in the pelvis. If it's very small, he'll know that there could be problems. Regardless, at each exam toward the end the effort will be made to guess the size of the baby.

Final determination, however, is often not known until transition is well under way.

Typically, unless it's known that the baby is very large compared to the pelvis, labor and transition will be allowed to continue. Drugs such as oxytocin or pitocin may be used to help. Under certain circumstances the doctor may decide to use forceps or vacuum extraction. The first uses a special tongs to grasp the baby. The second uses suction on top of the baby's head. Both techniques attempt to pull the baby down the birth canal. Neither is of much use if the CPD is beyond marginal. In such a case, a C-section will be needed.

The Operation

Unless the operation is performed as an emergency, you'll probably be allowed to attend. Normally, you'll be taken aside. While Mom is being prepared, you'll get into the sterile operating clothing needed to reduce the chances of infection. Her abdomen will be washed and sterilized. Depending on the situation, her pubic area may be shaved at least partially, usually across the top due to the nature of the incision. She will probably have an IV inserted into her arm. A catheter is used to keep the bladder empty.

In the past a general anesthetic was used. Today this is more rare. Most of the time the doctor will use an epidural. This blocks the pain while keeping the mother fully conscious. It also puts less stress on the infant and makes recovery for the mother far easier.

The incision is usually transverse—horizontal across the abdomen and just above the pubic area. This operation takes a little longer but brings with it many advantages. Cosmetically, the scar it leaves tends to be smaller and easier to hide. The risk of infection is decreased. Perhaps most important, with this kind of incision, it's quite possible that the mother can deliver vaginally the next time.

A midline (vertical) incision is faster, and may be used in a dire emergency when seconds count. Doing so cuts across the natural "grain" of the muscle and uterus. Healing afterward is more difficult, and leaves a weakened area. Because of this, if the woman becomes pregnant again, the doctor will almost certainly schedule a C-section. The danger of the uterus rupturing is too great.

The Premature or Undersized Baby

There are a number of reasons that the baby could be premature (earlier than thirty-six weeks). Usually it isn't a problem. If the baby is born exceptionally early, though, special care will be needed. Much the same is true of any baby less than five and one half pounds. It is treated as being premature, regardless of actual age.

The cause can sometimes be identified. Smoking, heavy drinking, drug use, physical trauma, certain diseases and infections, and other conditions are known to have connections to premature and undersized babies. If there is a multiple birth (twins, etc.), one might be much smaller than the other.

The amount of medical intervention varies, depending on the overall condition of the baby. Sometimes very little is needed. Other times the baby needs more extensive life support systems. A lot of it depends on the development of the lungs, with development of the heart and nervous system being a close second.

An incubator is often used. This provides a stable environment of about ninety degrees. Additional oxygen may be added, but usually won't be unless the infant is having problems with breathing.

The premature or underweight baby tends to be red, thin, and with a disproportionately large head. All are due to the fact that it hasn't completely matured. In the past many of these children died. Today steps can be taken. An infant born three full months early stands a good chance of survival.

The Late or Oversized Baby

Various conditions can cause the baby to become overly large (more than ten pounds). If it gets too large, delivery is going to be much more difficult—perhaps impossible unless a C-section is performed. This much is obvious. There are two other dangers. One is that the oversize baby could be crushing the umbilical cord. The other is that the placenta will age along with the baby. It begins to "shut down" and becomes less efficient. Also a time will come when abruption is more likely.

The doctor is unlikely to let the pregnancy last more than about two weeks beyond the predicted delivery date. If the baby is not oversize, it might be assumed that the original calculation was in error, but everything will be watched very closely.

Ultrasound will be used to help determine the size of the baby. This gives a fairly accurate idea of whether it is taking up too much room in the uterus, the amount of amniotic fluid, and also whether the baby will be too large for a vaginal birth. Ultrasound is also used for two other tests.

One measure is the *nonstress test* (NST). For this, ultrasound is used to measure fetal heart rate. The baby is monitored for about forty minutes. The goal is to see if the heart rate goes up when the baby moves. If it does, everything is probably normal. If the heart rate doesn't change, it could be an indication of trouble.

The *contraction stress test* (CST) requires contractions. For this reason it is kept for the woman already in labor. The test measures the baby's heart rate during a contraction. Ideally the heart rate should change very little, or not at all. If it does change, the combination of an overly large baby and the contraction could be squeezing the umbilical cord. If severe, the doctor may order a C-section. If mild, oxytocin or pitocin may be given to speed labor. Mom may also be encouraged to walk so that gravity can help.

After the birth, additional medical attention may or may not be needed. This depends on the reason the baby is large. If the cause is merely a long gestation, nothing additional will be needed. However, if the cause was something like gestational diabetes, the baby could be born diabetic, or more likely born with an overly high level of insulin.

Most of the problems are handled fairly easily, although the infant's condition may need to be monitored.

Multiple Birth

Having twins, triplets, or more isn't a "problem birth" as such. It does, however, often bring its own set of complications. With proper care, there is no reason that twins or triplets will make the pregnancy worse or dangerous. More than 90 percent are born healthy. Of the 10 percent that need additional help, most require only minimal medical attention. With three or more, the situation becomes more complicated.

In normal pregnancies (i.e., those not stimulated by fertility medications and procedures), twins result in about one out of a hundred cases. Triplets are more rare, with one such pregnancy out of about eight thousand pregnancies. One of each five hundred thousand pregnancies brings quadruplets. It's more likely for a woman to have a multiple pregnancy when she is in her thirties, if she has had a multiple pregnancy before, or if medical intervention is used to increase fertility.

A multiple birth is often detectable early in the pregnancy. The same test used to detect neural tube defects (see "The Doctors" in Chapter Seven) can indicate a multiple birth. Another indicator is when all the usual symptoms of pregnancy seem more severe. Later, ultrasound can be used to verify that she has a multiple pregnancy.

All the usual problems of pregnancy are likely to be amplified. Conditions such as preeclampsia are more common, and often more pronounced.

The birth itself is likely to cause a problem. A multiple birthing usually requires a C-section. The newborn infants are smaller than with a single birthing. As with any undersized baby, medical attention might be needed. In addition, birth defects occur at about double the usual percentage, which can require both short-term and long-term medical care.

The gestational period tends to be shorter. Twins often come at thirty-seven weeks, rather than the usual forty weeks. A woman carrying triplets often gives birth in the thirty-fifth week. About 10 percent of women who are carrying more than one child go into labor as early as twenty-eight weeks. This is another reason that twins, etc., are born smaller and less mature. They simply haven't had the time to finish prenatal growth.

A unique condition is the *twin-twin transfusion syndrome*. One of the twins gets an oversupply of blood, which causes the other to become anemic. This can also cause one to grow larger than the other. In both cases, if the difference between the two is severe, it may become necessary to induce birth early, or perhaps to perform a C-section.

Of special concern are identical twins. This happens when both develop from the same egg. Most of the time both develop just fine. However, in about three cases per hundred, the babies are inside the same amniotic sac. While this doesn't present a problem with their growth, the twins are moving around inside the same confined area. It's possible for the umbilical cords to become tangled. If this happens, the twins may die.

Blood Problems

There are four blood types—A, B, AB, and O. The person is also either Rh-positive (most people) or Rh-negative. The mother and baby are not necessarily in the same blood grouping. This doesn't usually cause major problems in a first pregnancy but could in later pregnancies.

If the baby's blood group is different from Mom's, her body could develop antibodies. If this happens and the next baby is also of a different blood grouping, the baby could develop anemia. Tests can be done, however. The effects of the mismatch can be minimized, such as by using Rh immune globulin (RhIg). This helps to reduce the buildup of antibodies.

If *You* Have to Deliver

It's unlikely, but possible, that you won't make it to the hospital, and that on the way you'll have to deliver. The most important thing to keep in mind at a time like that is that the vast majority of births go through to completion without any complications.

In *Emergency Childbirth,* by Dr. Gregory J. White—a manual written for laypeople who might find themselves in circumstances in which they have to deliver a baby (policemen, taxi drivers, etc.)—it says of the delivery doctor, "His simple tasks could have been performed by any bright eight-year-old."

The usual birth progresses and completes without intervention. With rare exception, a mother-to-be who is all alone will be able to successfully deliver her own baby. The assistant is there mostly to provide moral support. Secondarily he's there to assist what nature is already doing on its own, and has been for countless generations. Almost without exception, if there isn't time to get to the hospital, it's because the birth is progressing along lines that nature intended.

A complicated or difficult birth takes time. This in turn means that you will almost certainly have time to reach the hospital. Mom might suffer a bit, but all of you will make it.

Just in case, wash your hands before heading for the hospital. Better yet, take a complete shower and put on clean clothes. If you make it to the hospital—and you probably will—being clean for the birthing will make you feel better. If you have to stop along the way to make the delivery yourself, being clean is even more important.

On the drive to the hospital, slow down. It's far more dangerous to race or drive recklessly than it is to deliver the baby on the way.

If you have to stop to assist, your first concern should be for safety. Pull off to the side of the road and put on the flashers. Shut off the engine to eliminate fumes. Obviously, if it's cold outside, you may need to run the engine so that the heater will operate, but keep such running times to a minimum. However cold it is, open the windows at least an inch or two. With the windows closed the danger of carbon monoxide buildup is greatly increased.

Raising the hood is the traditional sign of your need for help. The first police officer who comes along will stop to see what help he or she can provide.

If there are many people around, quickly and efficiently find someone in the crowd to keep the others away. Mom doesn't need a crowd of curiosity seekers at such a time. Have someone else call for an ambulance.

Prepare yourself. Birth is messy. There is bound to be a fair amount of blood and other fluids, such as the amniotic fluid when the bag breaks. Seeing all this can cause panic in the uninitiated. Many people think that bleeding is automatically a sign of danger or pain. In giving birth, it's normal.

Also normal is the mother falling asleep between the contractions. She hasn't passed out, so don't panic. However, this is a good sign that the birth isn't going to be as immediate as you might have thought. You probably have time to get to the hospital.

Also be aware and prepared for Mom's reactions. As discussed in the last chapter, it's not at all uncommon for the woman to yell at her attendant. What you perceive an encouraging statement or attention could be irritating to her. Resist the urge to yell back at her. It won't help.

Preparation is important. A mother who expects pain and trouble will be much more difficult to calm than one who knows what is going on. Once she is giving birth, it's too late to educate her. In such a case, your calm attitude and encouraging remarks become even more important.

Encourage her to relax. Keep her well aware that someone who loves her is right at hand. No matter how hungry she might be, don't feed the mother at any time during the labor. Sips of water or ice chips are okay. Food is likely to come back up sooner or later, causing new complications of its own—including possible strangulation of the mother.

When it comes to medication, never, never, NEVER play doctor. Don't even give her aspirin to relieve the pain. (That won't work, anyway.) Certainly don't give her anything stronger. There have been cases in which a well-meaning father has given his wife puffs of marijuana (or something stronger) to relieve the pain, only to learn later that his home medicinal attempts will take years to repair—or that he is alone in the world.

Many experts say that no pain relief should be given even in a hospital. Even more realize that minimal attempts are okay *if* given under proper and professional care. You'd be hard-pressed to find anyone who has any valid knowledge who would advise the use of any drug without instant access to professional care.

Provide a clean surface for Mom. A classic emergency bedding is an unread newspaper. Lacking this, do the best you can, but be sure to have something clean and dry for wrapping the baby after the birth. Don't use up all the cloth you have.

For obvious reasons, she'll have to remove all clothing below the waist (with the exception of socks). Keep that clothing at hand, but try to keep it away from the site of the birth so that it doesn't become soiled or contaminated.

Do not have her undress from the waist up. After the baby is born, there will be plenty of time to put it to the mother's breast. Meanwhile, being covered eases the mother's sense of propriety, makes her feel less vulnerable, and also helps to keep her warm.

Then let nature and Mom do the job. If you're not sure what to do next, don't do anything at all. It's as simple as that. Depending on circumstances, you can pull over, help Mom get ready and into position, then start driving to the hospital again. (Again—drive carefully!)

Try not to touch the vagina, and certainly don't attempt to reach up inside. The birth canal is essentially sterile. By inserting your finger—such as to check the condition of the cervix (and do you *really* know what you're checking for?)—you're very possibly introducing contamination. That can only make matters worse. There is also the risk of causing physical damage to the mother or infant.

As the baby crowns, many women suddenly relax and stop pushing. Don't tell her to push. The end result could be a tearing of the tissues around the vulva and perineum. Keep in mind that a whole baby is trying to squeeze through the normally small opening. Time is needed for the tissues to stretch. And remember that when she does push, it should be *with* a contraction.

Don't pull on the baby. It will come on its own—or will

give you enough time to complete the drive to the hospital. As the baby comes, the most you should do is to cradle it out and prevent it from falling. Pulling on the head can easily cause permanent damage to the spinal cord. It can also cause nerve damage to the arms and can even damage or stop breathing.

In those rare circumstances when the shoulders are stuck, you can insert a finger to hook the underarm to assist in the delivery. Any such attempt is a last-ditch effort, however. Be sure to give plenty of time before you make it. If you have that time, you probably have time to get to the hospital.

It's possible that the baby's head will still be covered with membranes. This is one case in which the risk of infection takes second priority. Those membranes must be removed if the baby is to breathe. Most of the time, wiping the baby's face with a clean cloth will be enough. More rarely, the membrane will have to be physically torn clear.

You have probably seen movies or heard stories about spanking the newborn to get it to cry, and thus take a breath. DON'T! Doing this is useless and can injure the baby.

In the hospital the nurse will clear the nose and mouth with a special syringe and sterile cloth. You probably won't have either available, but do the best you can. Tilting the baby head-down will also help the fluid and mucus to drain.

Most of the time the baby will begin to cry all on its own in a minute or less. If the baby still hasn't taken a breath after a minute or two, artificial respiration may be necessary. Many childbirth classes and most hospitals teach infant and child CPR. This is important for all parents to know.

Basically, first clear the mouth. Place your mouth over the baby's tightly, and gently pinch the baby's nose closed. Puff a small amount of air into the baby's lungs. Count to about ten and repeat. Keep in mind that you are dealing with a newborn, not an adult. The puffs of air blown into the baby's mouth must be *very* gentle. Pump the baby's legs toward the chest about twelve times per minute. This action stimulates breathing.

A fairly common condition is to have the baby's neck wrapped in the umbilical cord. The instant reaction is to yank on it to keep the baby from strangling. Doing so is dangerous. Avoid touching the cord if at all possible, and certainly don't yank on it. Try to complete the birth, and only then gently unwrap the cord.

Don't cut the cord. There's no hurry. Leaving it attached for a while won't create problems. Cutting it too soon or incorrectly will. The cord is usually long enough to allow you to put the baby at the mother's breast, which will help deliver the afterbirth and reduce bleeding. As desirable as is a quick feeding, it doesn't take priority over the cord. If need be, simply place the baby on the mother's tummy and let the first feeding wait until medical professionals can take care of the cord.

Don't try to deliver the afterbirth. Chances are good that this will happen on its own, but that won't be for a while after the actual birth. Leaving it in place *can* cause problems, but nothing that can't be handled by the medical team at the hospital once you arrive. Trying to pull it out on your own will not only cause problems, it can kill the mother.

Bleeding accompanies the afterbirth. It can be considerable (as much as two cups) and can last for several minutes. Don't let this panic you unless there is a large gushing or the bleeding continues. If the bleeding is excessive, gently massage the tummy above the navel. Better yet, get to the hospital as quickly as possible. For that matter, once the baby is born, you've probably reached the end of the emergency and should again be on your way to the hospital.

If the placenta comes out, very carefully collect and set aside every part of it. This will be examined by the medical team to be sure that all of it came out. If pieces of it have remained inside, there can be serious complications.

Once the baby is out, keep both baby and mother warm,

even if that means giving up your shirt. Then, don't sit there along the side of the road and gloat. The time for jubilation will come later. Get to the hospital so that Mom and baby can be thoroughly checked out by professionals.

Once again, don't rush. What sense is there in saving one minute by running a red light, only to waste five explaining to an officer why you did it? Or worse, saving that minute only to get into a possibly fatal accident?

Staying calm at such a time isn't easy. It is critical that you do so. Force it on yourself. This is the single most important part you play. Your own calm appearance and demeanor will affect the mother just as much as will any panic you let show. The calmer you are, the calmer she will be. This will greatly reduce any possible problems during and after the birth.

SELF-DELIVERY IN BRIEF
❶ STAY CALM, no matter what
❷ Soothe and encourage the mother
❸ When in doubt, do nothing—don't play doctor
❹ Keep the field clean
❺ Keep the mother and baby warm
❻ Save all solids that pass from the mother's vagina
❼ Get medical attention as soon as possible

EMERGENCY KIT
Newspapers (unread)
Clean water
Clean blankets and other cloths
One or two flashlights
Syringe for baby's nose
Clean pan

12

Mom's Recovery

The length of time needed for recovery depends on how you define it. In one sense, Mom will have recovered well enough in a day or two to go home. Medically, the usual postpartum recovery period is said to be about six weeks, after which the doctor will want to see her again to be sure that all is well. More realistic is the old saying "Nine months in—nine months out." And of course, being pregnant changes her body for the rest of her life. Off on the fringe are those who claim that Mom never recovers. (Of course, they rarely bother to mention that giving birth reduces the incidence of a number of cancers and other ailments.)

The most critical time is the first week, and the first three days in particular. Most of the problems will show up during this period. With the growing practice of sending the mother home within twenty-four hours, it's important that you and she remain aware.

Chances are good that Mom will be feeling fairly normal before that first week is over. This doesn't mean that she is recovered. More weeks are needed. After six weeks, the healing will be complete, or close enough so the doctor can determine whether things are going well, or whether additional attention is needed.

The recovery period is usually uneventful. Other than helping Mom physically, there won't be much you can do. It's a time for healing, which means a time of patience.

Immediate Recovery

Immediately after the birth, Mom's body has just gone through quite an ordeal. She's likely to be sweaty and exhausted. Many women get the chills, or they might shiver while saying they are perfectly warm. Both are usually the result of the physical strain, and both will pass quickly. If not, the doctor or nurse should be notified. The same is true if she complains of dizziness, blurred vision, or a headache. All these symptoms will probably have a perfectly ordinary explanation. For example, some dizziness is normal simply because of what she has been through. It is to be expected even more so if she has had anesthetic. And in most cases, the mother will have medical care immediately on hand during this period.

It's explained in Chapter Ten, once the baby is born, the placenta (afterbirth) will come out easily and on its own, usually in an hour or less. It will be accompanied by uterine contractions. These are usually painless, to the point that Mom may not even notice. (Besides, she is probably exhausted from the delivery.)

It's possible that Mom was given oxytocin or pitocin during the labor. It's also possible that she will be given one of these drugs to encourage the afterbirth. This is one medical reason that the mother is often encouraged to breast-feed right away. Breast-feeding stimulates the natural production of oxytocin. Almost miraculously, oxytocin also reduces bleeding.

Many women report a feeling of exhilaration. This may come immediately after the birth, or after she is finally allowed to sit up. When finally taken to the recovery room (or just left alone if in an LDR), she may have trouble getting to sleep—and if she does, may have trouble staying asleep for long. It's not at all unusual for the attending father to sleep faster, deeper, and longer.

The First Days

Assuming that all has gone well—and it usually does—after an hour or so, you and Mom will be left alone at last. The doctor may recommend or even require (depending on the conditions) that the baby be taken to the nursery. One reason is so the staff can give the baby a much more thorough examination. The other is to allow the mother to rest. However, it is becoming more and more common for the baby to "room in," which is to say that the baby and parents stay together.

There will be a steady flow of nurses coming in to make sure that things are as they should be. Exactly what happens depends on the circumstances. This could be anything from the nurse checking blood pressure and asking, "How are you feeling?" to more extensive medical intervention.

The doctor may or may not stop by. In most cases there is little need of this, other than as a courtesy and to build a sense of security. He will be informed if anything requires his attention, however. In other words, don't be concerned or feel slighted if he doesn't come in. There is usually no need for the visit.

Bleeding during the birth and afterbirth is normal. It's also normal in the beginning stages of recovery. During the first three or four days, the vaginal discharge, called *lochia*, tends to be fairly heavy and dark red. Lochia is made of blood, mucus, and uterine lining. At first, as healing begins, there will be more blood in it, and a heavier flow. The flow should steadily decrease as healing takes place. It should also become more pink rather than red. Eventually it will become clear, and finally return to normal in both color and flow, eventually ceasing.

It may be unpleasant, but make it a point to find out if the flow is normal. One reason is so you can spot potential dangers. The other is that you may have spotted a problem just in asking.

Bleeding is normal—hemorrhage is not. It's possible that all seemed well immediately after the birth, only for a vein or artery to open hours or days later. If you make it a point to find out what is considered "normal," especially in the quantity, you'll be better able to detect hemorrhage. You'll also be able to avoid panic, thinking that a normal flow is something more serious.

Those first days are the most critical, because this is when hemorrhage is most common. Once again, this is why it is important to become familiar with what is normal. Hemorrhage is rarely immediately fatal, but is definitely a sign that something has to be done quickly—and perhaps immediately.

If the flow seems to be subsiding and becoming more pink, then increases, turns more red—or if there is a strong odor, and especially if there are any solid chunks of tissue—contact the doctor.

The First Weeks

Once the exhilaration has worn off, Mom is likely to feel a little (or a lot) beat up. This usually fades after a week or two of steady improvement. There is no real standard or guideline. If the mother was in decent physical condition, and took care of herself during the pregnancy—if there were no complications during the birthing—she should be feeling better and better as the days go by. It may surprise you just how quickly this happens.

There will be a very quick weight loss of about thirteen to fifteen pounds. This comes from the rather sudden removal of the baby, the amniotic fluid, and the placenta. It's common, and normal, for the mother to urinate frequently. Her body is quite naturally getting rid of fluids that have built up in her body during the pregnancy.

After the quick loss of weight, the remaining loss should be slow and steady. This is not the time for Mom to be in a hurry or to diet. Especially if she is breast-feeding, and even if not, a sound, balanced diet is important. Weight loss will come on its own, naturally, and should not be forced.

If she has had an episiotomy or tearing of the tissues, the surgical site is very likely to itch. The doctor may suggest a local anesthetic, such as Americaine. She may even be "given" a spray can of an anesthetic at the hospital. This is also readily available at any drugstore, and at half the cost, or less. Local anesthetics such as these are available in spray cans, ointments, and sometimes as a liquid.

It also helps if she has a wash bottle to spray water on the vaginal area after urination. Urine has a salt content, which can sting and irritate the healing wound. The washing relieves this. So does the coolness of the water. More important, though, is that this helps keep the area clean, which helps prevent any infection.

These same steps help to relieve other problems. Most women have hemorrhoids after giving birth. These can be minor or extremely painful. It's possible that the doctor noticed them after the birthing and already took surgical steps to relieve the condition.

The help for episiotomy, tissue tearing, and hemorrhoids is all pretty much the same. Ice packs are often recommended for cooling. Medicated pads, such as Tucks, help clean and cool. Sitz baths are used to promote cleanliness. In some cases the doctor may suggest heat-lamp treatments, especially if the area needs help in keeping dry.

There won't be much you can do other than to provide emotional support, and to make sure that all the needed supplies are always on hand. This includes pads such as she'd use during a normal period. (She should not be using tampons at this time.)

It's not unusual for her to experience episodes of sudden heavy sweating. These are more common at night. In almost every case they mean nothing other than that her body is struggling to return to normal. Cool to tepid showers can help. At this point, however, baths are still to be avoided.

These bouts could last several weeks. If they continue, don't be too concerned but at least notify the doctor. If they are accompanied by fever, anything even remotely resembling convulsions, or even headaches, don't wait. There is probably nothing wrong. Or she might have an infection that needs to be treated. There is the distant chance that something more serious is happening. Be especially alert if there is bleeding.

In the previous section, bleeding and hemorrhage were discussed. Once again, bleeding is normal in the first days. It should decrease, turn pink, then clear and finally stop. If it doesn't stop, or if it increases, becomes more bloody, don't wait to contact the doctor. This is a fairly rare situation, but is one that must be taken very seriously.

Also common are constipation and difficulty in urination. These have both physical and psychological factors.

The entire region from the top of the pubic area to the top of the anus is likely to be sore. So may be the muscles that assist in going to the bathroom. The almost-always-present hemorrhoids can make it painful before, during, and in trying to clean afterward. It's very possible that the soreness might skyrocket while she's on the toilet and could continue for some time after.

Whether or not she has had an episiotomy or tissue tearing, there could be a fear in her mind—even if she doesn't recognize it herself—that additional damage could be done. She might be afraid of opening the stitches or causing other harm.

Julia had just such a problem. Going to the bathroom hurt. She began holding back, to delay the pain. Eventually she began to eat and drink less. All of this had an effect on her general condition. She developed constipation, lost weight, and finally got a bladder infection.

Once again, there isn't much you can do other than to give emotional support. You can encourage her to wash afterward rather than wipe. You might even consider installing a showerhead on a long hose to make this easier, if you don't already have one. Also be sure that there is plenty of fruit and fiber in her diet (and yours). For example, bringing her slices of apple as you relax together in the evening is a nice treat that will be tasty and can help relieve constipation.

Be aware, however, that difficulty in relieving herself might have a physical reason. Infections of the urinary tract are fairly common. Throughout pregnancy and after, the bladder may not empty. In addition, after the birth her body is, by nature, trying to get rid of all the fluids built up during the pregnancy. She will have an increased need to urinate, but may be physically hampered to do so. Trapped urine increases the chances of an infection. The usual initial symptoms are a difficulty in urination accompanied by a burning sensation. If caught early enough, these infections are usually treated fairly easily.

Along with constipation may come gas. This is particularly common with women who have had a C-section. Remember that the digestive system changed during the pregnancy, slowed during labor, and eventually stopped. Now it has to return to normal again.

For her sake, at least for now, avoid foods that are hard to digest. Keep beans, spicy foods, even dairy products to a minimum. Walking and other light exercise can also help. In fact, these can help in many ways.

Generally, exercise in the first days should be minimal. You can be a big help by handling the cleaning, vacuuming, mopping, etc. As recommended in Chapter Four, if you've prepared meals for several days and put them in the freezer, and if you've helped keep the house clean as the time for delivery approached, that first week at home will be simple and enjoyable. Even with this, spend a little extra effort during those first weeks home. It might mean getting up a little earlier so that some of the chores are done before you leave for work, but it can also be fun.

As time goes by, she'll be able to handle more and more. Don't baby her *too* much. The exercise will do her good. Just be careful that the exercise isn't too strenuous. This is not yet the time for her to help carry fifty-pound bags of dog food or to do any heavy lifting.

C-section Recovery

Most things that can be said about recovery for a woman who has delivered vaginally are true for those who had a C-section. Other conditions are different.

This begins with a longer stay in the hospital. A C-section is a common operation, and a relatively safe one. Even so, *any* operation can bring problems. Typically she will spend up to a week in the hospital afterward, mostly to be sure that she is okay and that no infection sets in. Remember that the incision has cut through the skin, through the muscle, and through the uterus. All this has to be stitched together afterward and then has to heal.

During the first few days of recovery, Mom will be

watched carefully. The incision, and her body in general, will probably be cleaned with a sponge bath. After a few days she may be allowed to shower, although she may need assistance.

She will be encouraged to move about in the bed right from the start. This will be difficult for her, and perhaps painful, but it's important. If you are there, be encouraging. She is going through a lot, even with the painkillers.

It's true that the woman who has had a C-section won't have the episiotomy or torn perineal tissues. Even in the worst of these, a topical anesthetic is usually enough, with a mild oral analgesic needed only rarely. The incision for a C-section is more serious. A much heavier anesthetic is needed to perform the operation.

At one time it was common practice to use a general anesthetic, which means that the mother is made unconscious. This presents a greater risk to both the mother and child, however, and extends the time needed for recovery. The woman is likely to experience dizziness and nausea, possibly for several days.

Today other methods are used when possible. The mother is usually fully conscious during the operation. Even so, the entire area is made numb. Afterward this anesthetic is removed, and painkillers are used instead. Some fairly potent painkillers may be needed for a while. Care is taken in prescribing and administering these, especially if the mother is breast-feeding.

Some women try to "wean" themselves off the painkillers quickly. Unless she is suffering or unable to sleep, there is rarely a need to be concerned about this. The opposite is not true. If she is taking too many painkillers, there are a number of potential dangers for both the mother and a breast-fed child.

As has been said so many times in this book, don't try to play doctor. It could be that the painkillers aren't effective. The doctor can switch her to another, or may recommend a higher dose. He may want to see her, to make sure that something else isn't wrong. These painkillers are for wounds that are healing, not for problems that may be occurring that cause increased pain. It could also be simply that her pain threshold is low.

Once she is home, all the same "rules" apply as with a vaginal birth. She needs time to heal. Light exercise is both okay and beneficial, but heavy exercise can cause trouble. At the same time, lack of exercise can also bring on problems. Even if she merely walks around a little, that will help. It will help keep muscle tone, help the wound to heal faster, and is one of the best things she can do to reduce flatulence, which is so common in C-section patients.

Expect her to be reluctant. Even mild exercise such as walking can hurt. She may need your encouragement.

The need for your help around the house increases. Again, mild exercise is of benefit, but after this operation she is prone to fatigue and exhaustion. A part of this comes from the painkillers. These can make her feel sleepy. They can also make her feel a little too good, which can lead her to do too much too soon.

For most women, this proceeds with relative ease. There will be pain, of course. It's likely that the wound will itch. An anesthetic cream may be recommended by the doctor. Help her to be aware of redness, and especially of any signs of pus around the wound. This indicates an infection. If the incision is kept clean, the chances of infection are greatly reduced. Regardless, most infections are easily treated with antibiotics. (Some doctors prescribe these routinely.)

A problem unique to C-section is that the mother may feel that she somehow failed as a woman. If she had her heart set on delivering vaginally, having a C-section can make her feel cheated, even angry. She might blame herself, the doctor, the nurse, or you.

As stated in Chapter Eleven, although some believe that doctors resort to C-section too quickly, and although this *could* be the truth in your case, there are times when the operation is necessary. It has nothing to do with her ability as a woman or mother. And it doesn't necessarily mean that she can't deliver vaginally the next time.

Other than in emergencies, most C-sections performed use an incision with the muscle and tissue rather than against them. Healing is more complete this way, and there is far less chance of rupture later during a second birthing. VBAC (vaginal birth after C-section) is becoming more and more common.

Breast-feeding

Most problems with breast-feeding disappear after a couple of weeks. Time is needed for both the mother and baby to learn how. Time is needed for her breasts to adjust. This period of adjustment tends to go faster if the mother has had children before, and has breast-fed them, but even then some time is needed.

Even if she isn't breast-feeding, her breasts will secrete colostrum for several days. (This secretion may have started before the birth.) Then regular milk starts. Nature has again taken a hand in things. Colostrum is the perfect food for the newborn, and the milk is perfect for the growing newborn.

The breasts will also probably adapt to the demand. As the child grows and needs more, the amount of milk produced increases. Even with twins or more, it's possible for her breasts to adapt and produce enough for all.

Obviously, sometimes there are problems. Julie had two children, four years apart. She breast-fed both, and each time, despite her best efforts and a balanced diet, after about a month her breasts weren't producing enough milk. She had to supplement with formula and very soon abandoned the effort to breast-feed entirely.

Other women suffer from various conditions in the

breast, such as mastitis (infection of the breast). This can be painful, and can also reduce or prevent her ability to breast-feed, and usually requires medical attention.

Breast engorgement is fairly normal. Mom begins to produce milk. It often takes a while for the amount produced to match the needs of the baby. If too much is produced, the breasts grow larger, often get harder, and may even become lumpy both in appearance and to the touch. It is also common for Mom to feel that her breasts are warm and tingly. It can be painful, and might even lead Mom and you to think she has mastitis.

Usually engorgement decreases after a few days. Meanwhile, cool cloths can help, as can a good support bra. A common mistake many make is to attempt to relieve the situation by massage or by using a breast pump. While this can provide temporary relief, the end effect will be the opposite of what is needed. Both stimulate milk production, at a time when what is needed is a reduction.

Mastitis shows itself in a different way. Bacteria makes its way inside the breast, usually through cracks in the nipple. Infection sets in and could spread. As with other infections, it's likely to show itself as warm areas on the breast (usually beneath) that may also be reddish in color. She will likely have a temperature. Common advice is that if her temperature rises above 100.4° F, she should see the doctor. If she has an infection, he will probably prescribe antibiotics. Be aware that this can change the color and appearance of the baby's bowel movements, but is believed to be safe.

The doctor will usually recommend that she continue to breast-feed. Another suggestion he might give is for her to breast-feed more often but for shorter periods. Both help to keep the breasts empty and more comfortable.

Yet another possibility, and one that is fairly common, is for a milk duct to clog. This can usually be felt with the fingers, and can sometimes be seen visually. At times it can become painful for the mother. The condition will often fix itself. A warm cloth may help. Unfortunately, the condition can also lead to infection. Don't wait too long to seek a doctor's help.

Postpartum Depression

It might be surprising to learn how common it is for the new mother to feel depressed. You'd think she would be thrilled and happy. All the complaints of pregnancy are over, as is the pain of giving birth. There is a new baby in your lives. The world should be bright and cheery!

This isn't always the case. Many women feel mild and occasional depression after the birth—so many that it is considered to be normal and natural. When mild, most refer to it as "the baby blues." Up to 80 percent of all women feel this. A more serious case is postpartum depression, or PPD. PPD affects somewhere between 10 and 20 percent, depending on how the diagnosis is made and defined. The worst case, called postpartum psychosis, is rare.

Her body has gone through months of changes, culminating in the ordeal of giving birth, and during recovery is struggling to return to normal. Her hormones and everything else are trying to adjust. She is tired, even if she doesn't know it. She is also likely to be in pain. She might be disappointed in how the pregnancy and birthing went. For example, she might have been determined to use no drugs but ended up having to ask for anesthetic. Or she might have been set on delivering "naturally," but a C-section was necessary.

She could have been dreaming of breast-feeding and has found that, for some reason, she can't. Like you, she might have concerns about caring for the baby, and raising the child. Will she be a good mother? Will you be a good father? Will the child be troublesome? What about all the expenses?

Beyond all this, a very exciting event is now over. Months

passed between her finding that she was pregnant and the birth. All that time, she was the center of attention. The birth itself was a goal to be reached, and anticipated. Now it's over.

It's somewhat like the child looking forward to Christmas. Decorations go up all around town. At school there are Christmas plays and other activities. The parents have gone shopping for the presents. They're hidden around the house and are not to be seen until Christmas. Santa is coming to bring even more presents. The tree goes up—and so does the child's sense of anticipation. The night before Christmas, the level of excitement is so high that many children have a hard time going to sleep. Then comes Christmas morning, with all those bright packages. Within a short time, however, the last package has been opened. It's over.

It doesn't take a selfish child to feel the let-down. You've probably felt this way yourself. It's perfectly normal. The anticipation is part of the magic.

The same is true with pregnancy. Now that it's over, the anticipation is gone, and the work of feeding and raising the child begins. It's not that Mom is disappointed, but the whole situation has suddenly changed.

Incidentally, although it's almost never discussed or even mentioned, fathers can suffer from the same things. Although your body hasn't gone through all the physical changes, the emotional changes that you *have* faced, and still do, are almost exactly the same as hers. There are support groups all across the country for women, as well as national organizations. Nothing like this exists for the new father. This will be covered in more depth in Chapter Fifteen (and will be mentioned in Chapter Sixteen, a chapter for Mom to help her understand what *you* are going through).

One of the best tools against depression is to be sure Mom doesn't get fatigued. If she is rested, healing proceeds more quickly and she feels better in general. The simple fact that you are allowing her to rest by doing more of the household chores, and that you are being a full part of this, can be tremendously uplifting.

Anxiety is another symptom. Sometimes she can pinpoint what is worrying her—other times she just has the sense of worry. How you handle this depends on the situation. There is no perfect advice that works every time. For example, you might relieve her anxiety by being cheerful. If she sees you cheerful and positive, she might follow. Other times, however, this can make things worse.

Be supportive, but also be aware. It's possible that the baby blues have progressed to become PPD, which could progress into psychosis. The time may come (but probably won't) that medical help is needed. It's also possible that there is a physical cause rather than emotional. This is another case of *don't play doctor.*

Accept that mild depression is normal—for both of you. Anxiety is also normal. Most of the time these things disappear on their own. This will happen more quickly if fatigue is avoided, and if you each support the other.

Sex

It is generally inadvisable to have intercourse anytime during the six-week recovery period. The actual amount of time could be longer, depending on circumstances and the results of the postpartum examination.

The wait doesn't bother most men. Not only are there other ways for sexual release, the truly involved father will be just as exhausted in those first weeks as the mother. In interviews a fairly common "complaint" among new mothers was that the father seemed more interested in the child than in her, and seemed to be having *no* problem with abstinence. One woman joked that her husband was so willing to wait that she wondered if he was being unfaithful. (The comments were invariably made half-jokingly. Those who had husbands who were involved were thrilled.)

However you feel, intercourse too soon can be dangerous. At the very first, it will be painful for her, and brings the danger of opening wounds and/or causing infection. Even when it *seems* safe, these dangers may still exist.

Also be aware that many women have fears about resuming intercourse after giving birth. This is nothing against you, so don't take it personally. Relax. Be patient.

There is a common misbelief that a new mother, and again especially a breast-feeding mother, can't become pregnant. This isn't true. The chances of her getting pregnant again are considerably lower than normal, usually for several months, especially if she is breast-feeding. This doesn't mean that she *can't* get pregnant, only that she is less likely to. Don't trust the statistics, or rely on her breast-feeding as a form of contraception. You just might find yourselves becoming parents again sooner than expected.

Most physicians recommend that the mother have a period of some months to fully recover from a birth before considering another pregnancy. For that matter, most women would prefer a break between.

Possible Problems

One of the most dangerous complications, hemorrhage, has been mentioned. Infection of healing wounds and incisions was also mentioned, as were urinary tract infections. Each has to do with the recovery process and being aware of it. Three potential problems, however, are not so visible.

The problem of preeclampsia (high blood pressure) has been discussed many times in this book. Usually it disappears within three days after the birth. Occasionally it gets worse and can develop into full eclampsia. As has been said before, there are often no symptoms, which is why the doctor pays such close attention to her blood pressure throughout the pregnancy. In most cases, if there is a potential problem, it will have been spotted. Most women who continue to have a problem with this condition had a serious problem with it during the pregnancy. It's extremely rare for a woman who has been fine all along to suddenly develop eclampsia after the birth. Normally you don't have to be worried unless this is the case, and/or she didn't take care of herself during the pregnancy.

Although preeclampsia has few or no symptoms, eclampsia can have some that are very alarming. There might be pain on the right side of the abdomen. She might have headaches, or see flashes of light. In rare cases she might have seizures or drop into unconsciousness.

Less than 10 percent of the time, the woman will develop an internal infection of the uterus. This is called *endometritis*. Most of these cases occur after a C-section. Other possible causes are a very long labor or if the amniotic membranes broke well before the birth. With all of these conditions, bacteria can get into the uterus and begin to multiply.

Most of the time this kind of infection will show itself within two or three days of the birth. Even when this infection takes place, it is usually fairly mild and easy to control. That doesn't mean it should be ignored. Sometimes it requires hospitalization, with antibiotics administered through an IV drip.

Common symptoms include fever (usually low), headache, backache, and loss of appetite. She may begin to feel contractions again. Her abdomen might be sensitive. If the infection has set in well, the vaginal discharge (which is normal, remember) could have a bad odor. Note that all of these symptoms can represent many other things—some simple, some serious. Left untreated, the infection can spread to surrounding organs and tissues.

The change in hormones can cause blood clotting.

Thrombophlebitis, for example, is a condition in which clots form in the legs or pelvic region. This reduces circulation in the area, and can often be quite painful. More dangerous, the clots can break loose. If they do and move into the lungs or heart, the result is potentially fatal.

Fortunately, this condition is rare. Those at risk will probably have been diagnosed as such during the pregnancy. Medications such as blood thinners might be used. In a severe case, which is even more rare, she might have to stay in the hospital.

What Can You Do?

Even if you can't be there all the time, there are many things you can do. Preparation will help. (Read Chapter Four). If you're unprepared, there are many simple but nutritious meals possible even for someone who has never cooked before. Keep in mind that it should be well balanced, high in fiber, low in fat, and that she needs plenty of liquids. The other chores—cleaning, washing the clothes and dishes—aren't a strain unless you make them that way.

Mom needs rest for at least a few days. A week isn't too long, if you remember that she also needs mild to moderate exercise. She will have the tendency to grab catnaps while the baby sleeps. Friends and relatives, even those who know this, could be calling. If you don't already have one, consider getting an answering machine, set to answer on the first ring. Have her turn this on and unplug the phone when she rests. Those calls can be returned later.

In general, indulge her for two or three weeks. She deserves it, and needs it. This can also help develop an important bonding for you.

13

Dealing with the Newborn

*H*aving a new baby in the house is going to be one of the biggest changes you will ever experience. (If you already have children, you know what I mean.) You might have thought that getting married was a major change. It was. *This* change is even more intense. A wife can take care of herself. She can get a drink of water if she is thirsty, make a sandwich if she is hungry, or tell you if she is sick or wants something. A baby can't do any of that.

For the first few years, the child is totally dependent on you and the mother. The time will come when the child wants—demands!—more independence. This will begin sooner than you might believe. The so-called terrible twos are aptly named. By then the child has learned to walk and to speak. The proverbial wings are being stretched, but with some frustration attached due to natural, and imposed, restrictions.

After that come the years of growth, then the teenage years, perhaps college, marriage—and before you know it, you'll be a grandfather, holding yet another generation in your arms. It all happens very fast.

For now, you have something of more immediate concern. You are a father. Whether this is your first child, your second, or your tenth, there is a new and unique individual in your lives—one who needs you. Although the child may not show it in obvious ways for a while, those needs go well beyond the physical. Keep in mind that there is strong evidence that the newborn can already recognize the mother, and often the father, immediately after the birth. This continues to grow, both over the coming months and over the coming years.

The foundation, both physical and mental, begins here.

The New Baby

Although it varies over a wide range, at birth the average baby weighs about seven to eight pounds and is twenty inches long. Its head is about one third as large as all the rest of the baby, giving it a very distinctive top-heavy appearance. The head will usually be about the same diameter as the chest. The arms and legs will seem short—almost stubby. The body will give the appearance of being quite long in comparison. It will take some years before the usual proportion of head to body comes about.

As you know, the bones of the baby's skull move. This allows passage through the pelvic outlet and down the birth canal. It also means that the baby's head is likely to have an odd shape. The longer the labor, the more molding is likely. This elongation almost always disappears in a matter of days. You'll probably see a change within just a few hours.

In addition, actual damage might have resulted from the birth. Bumps on the head, for example, are quite common.

(One doctor announced to the new parents, "Your child is already a little devil. He has two horns.") This is called *cephalohematoma* and is caused by slight rupturing of the blood vessels beneath the baby's scalp brought on by the baby's head being bumped and crushed against the pelvic bones of the mother.

The condition is rarely of concern. It might cause a slight elevation in the chances of the baby getting jaundice (also rarely of any real concern and quite common). If severe enough, it might take a number of years before the bumps disappear completely, but regardless of how bad they seem to you, they aren't hurting your baby.

Some babies are born covered with a white coating called vernix, which gives the baby a ruddy appearance. If there is no vernix, it's possible that the baby went beyond term. A yellow vernix is a sign of fetal distress and sometimes post-maturity. There is nothing you can do about this, but it gives the medical staff clues about other conditions that might arise.

The attending nurse will clean away most or all of the vernix. What remains is likely to peel shortly after the birth *(desquamation)*. It can look like peeling skin after a sunburn, but it doesn't hurt the child.

The skin itself may have small white bumps similar in appearance to white pimples. This is *milia* and is rarely of concern. Leave them alone and they'll go away on their own. Red bumps *(macules)* also common, and are also of little concern.

The genitals are often large and swollen, particularly with male babies. The ears and nose are likely to be flattened. It's fairly common for the eyes to be puffy and have small red spots. This condition is called *conjunctuval hemorrhage* and is rarely dangerous. It's caused by strains on the blood vessels during the birthing. All of these will disappear in time. Usually the ears come out within a day or two. The nose follows. The swelling of the eyes and nose, and red spots in the eyes, could take a week or two.

The baby's eyes are almost always a blue or gray in color. The pigments that give the actual color won't develop for a while. It may be several months before you know what your baby's true eye color is. So if both you and your wife have brown eyes, and your baby is born with blue eyes, it means nothing.

Nonwhite infants often get dark bluish spots, somewhat like bruises and particularly in the area of the buttocks. They are called *Mongolian spots* but have nothing at all to do with the birth defect Down's syndrome, formerly called mongolism, and they are not a problem.

The First Tests and Exams

The baby's first exam takes place just moments after birth. The baby is examined both visually and by touch. Even the fingers and toes are counted. The baby is then weighed and measured. Both numbers are critical and will be used during the first months of the baby's life to determine how well it is growing.

The Apgar test is given at one minute, then repeated at five minutes. As discussed in Chapter Ten, this test helps determine the baby's overall condition. Breathing, muscle tone, response to stimulation, heart rate, and skin color each earn a score from zero (the worst) to two (the best), resulting in an overall score of zero (extreme emergency) to ten (the rare perfect score).

It's not unusual for the baby to be limp immediately after the birth. This can frighten the parents, because it can seem that the child isn't alive. This changes rapidly, however, with the first cry. Poor muscle tone after five minutes, or a poor score in any of the areas, can be a bad sign. It indicates that medical intervention might be needed.

The skin color and flexibility will be watched. These are indicators of many things. It's not unusual for the baby to come out bluish. As with the limpness, this can frighten new parents into thinking that their baby has died. But within a very short time the blue should disappear, with the skin turning a healthy tone. This shows that the circulatory and respiratory systems are functioning. (Be aware that the fingers and toes might remain bluish for a while longer, but this normally goes away in a day or two.)

If the proper skin tone doesn't come right away, even more attention will be paid to breathing and air passages. *Cyanosis,* the blue tone from lack of oxygen, can be caused by blocked passages.

If the baby is pale, it could indicate circulatory failure and/or shock. It could also be caused by a respiratory obstruction, cerebral anoxia, narcosis (drug-related problems, including unconsciousness or stupor), or adrenal failure. In many cases, a pale baby is worse than a blue baby.

The skin tone will be examined. Most babies have wrinkled skin. This is normal and goes away quickly. The doctors and nurses will be concerned, however, if the skin is overly wrinkled. Among other things, this could be a sign that the baby is dehydrated, usually caused by poor maternal diet. It can also be caused by toxemia in the mother, a defective placenta, or some kind of infection. In most cases, the problem can be solved (if it is recognized).

A symptom of jaundice is a yellowing of the skin and of the whites of the eyes. Even if all seems well, the nurse will press a thumb against the baby's forehead. This shouldn't yellow. It should return to the normal skin color very quickly in any case. In most cases, mild jaundice is common and no problem. Bilirubin forms in the skin, caused by the breakdown of an excess of red blood cells. (It is also caused, in all people, by the breakdown of old red blood cells.) Usually the liver is able to get rid of the bilirubin, but in a newborn the liver isn't mature enough.

Usually all that is needed is to expose the baby's skin to bright light. This helps stimulate the natural skin pigments and reduces the bilirubin content. You might even hear that your new baby needs "bilirubin treatment," which is this kind of exposure. The doctor may recommend that you continue to do this, such as by letting the child be in the sunlight for a few minutes each day. Frequent nursings and giving additional water may also help.

The condition will be watched, however. It could be a symptom of an infection or other medical problem. Jaundice within the first twenty-four hours can indicate an infection, or perhaps either an Rh or ABO blood incompatibility. The last two are far more common if the mother has had previous children. Left untreated, any of these three can create complications, both immediate and in the future. Treated, further difficulties are rare.

Very common is "psychological jaundice," also called "third-day jaundice." This appears usually between the third and seventh days. It is rarely of any concern, but bears watching. If it occurs after the fifth day, it could indicate a medical problem.

"Breast-milk jaundice" is far more infrequent and shows usually between the second and third weeks. Once again, there is rarely much need for concern. Contact with the doctor is important, of course, but chances are good that the worst scenario is that Mom may have to stop breast-feeding for a few days.

Another visual exam will be for birthmarks (*hemangiomas*). Part of this is for identification. These marks might be present at birth, or could appear at any time during the first year or even beyond. The vast majority mean nothing at all. A few are a sign of something more dangerous. (Any time a blemish appears for no known reason, and especially one that changes in shape or color, a doctor should have a look.)

The baby will be checked for signs of edema. Some swelling is normal. The genital area is often swollen. Of greater concern is swelling that is pretty much limited to the hands and feet. This could be a sign of neonatal tetanus. This same condition can be caused later by an infection of the stump where the umbilical cord was cut.

Baby's First Days Home

The day will come when you will leave the hospital and go home as a family. Especially if this is your first child, going home can be scary. Now you're on your own.

Some have said that the baby's entire life at first is made up of nothing but eating and sleeping. That's not only inaccurate, it's misleading. Even a newborn baby will have periods of activity and alertness. It will kick and squirm and even look around. If the baby actually does nothing but eat and sleep, it might be time to see the doctor, especially if the baby doesn't even seem to want to wake for feeding. (See "Warning Signs and Illnesses," in this chapter.)

The baby should urinate about twenty-four hours after the birth. In roughly two days he or she should pass the first bowel movement. The material passed is called *meconium*. It looks a little like black tar and has little or no odor. If this doesn't come after the third day, the doctor should be called. There is probably no cause for concern, but he may wish to examine the child, just in case.

After this, the stools can be light or dark, although usually they are light. A baby that is being breast-fed will tend to have stools that are looser, softer, more yellow, and with less odor. The volume, frequency, and odor will all increase. You may get the idea that you're spending half of your day changing diapers, but keeping the baby clean and dry is important.

The healthy baby will already have the ability to react. For example, if you touch its cheek, it will turn in search of food (the nipple). This is called the rooting reflex. The sucking reflex will cause the baby to begin sucking, even if all that is found is your finger. Also, if you touch the baby's palm, it will close its fingers (the grasping reflex).

The baby hasn't yet learned fear, or a fear reaction, but instinctually the body will tighten and the arms and legs will jump if there is a loud noise (such as a clap). This is the *Moro reflex*.

A shock to some parents is when the baby exhibits certain adult female characteristics. For example, it's possible that a newborn girl will have what seems to be a period. A girl *or* boy may have a leaking of milk from the nipples. These things are not of concern and will fade in time. They are caused by the baby having hormones in its system from the mother. (Bleeding, however, should *always* be checked by a qualified doctor.)

It's a fair chance that the baby will already react to at least the mother's voice, and possibly yours, too. If not, this will come quickly. Within a short time many babies become so attached that they will begin to cry if held by a stranger, and calm immediately when taken by someone familiar.

Especially if this is your first child, expect it to take a while before you learn to find what is making the baby cry. Crying is normal, and often the baby's only way to communicate. (It also helps the baby develop the respiratory system.) Accept that there is always a reason for it. The baby might be hungry, have gas, be cold or too warm, needs a diaper change, has a rash. . . . It might also be that the baby is sick.

Those first days can be frightening because you can't always tell what is making the baby cry. Give it time. You'll learn.

Feeding

Some newborns will suckle for long periods. Others will suckle for just a few minutes at a time. Just be sure that baby is getting enough. (He'll usually let you know.) The spacing between the feedings will gradually lengthen in the coming months. At the very first, feeding is needed about every two hours. Making it more exhausting, this isn't like dealing with someone older. You cannot schedule the meals. When baby is hungry, *baby is hungry!* If it's 2:00 A.M. and you're tired, baby doesn't care.

If Mom is breast-feeding, most of the job will fall to her. This doesn't mean you can't help out. One obvious way is for her to express breast milk and store it in the refrigerator. That way you can take some of the feedings. Another option is to use baby formula for those feedings.

It will also help if you take on a few more of the household chores. Sometimes all that's needed is to sit with her while she feeds the baby. This is a great time for sharing, and for letting her know that she's not alone.

For thousands of years the newborn was either breast-fed—or starved. There were no other options, no baby formula. Today all this has changed. In almost every case it will be recommended that the mother breast-feed. This is not only less expensive, it helps the baby's immune system. However, there are times when the mother can't breast-feed.

There are many possible reasons for this. It could simply be that the mother doesn't want to. Also, especially at first, breast-feeding can hurt—and can hurt later when the baby develops those first sharp little teeth. (In such cases, a compromise might be for her to express the milk and feed the baby from a bottle.) There are various illnesses that make breast-feeding difficult or impossible. Some, which require medication, mean that it could be dangerous for the baby to receive the milk. Such conditions may be temporary or permanent.

In Chapter Four it was recommended that you have at least *some* baby formula in the house, and learn how to use it. Don't expect there to be plenty of warning for its need.

There probably will be, but don't count on it. By having a small quantity on hand, you're ready.

One new father, for example, thought he was all prepared the day his wife went to visit her sister and left him home alone with the baby. She'd expressed milk the night before and earlier that morning. The two bottles were in the refrigerator, ready to go. A few hours after she left, the baby began to cry. He cuddled his new daughter as the milk warmed on the stove. She took to it hungrily and was soon satisfied.

A while later, she was hungry again. Feeling confident, he lifted his daughter from the crib, went to the kitchen, opened the refrigerator door, reached for the bottle of milk—and promptly dropped it on the floor. His wife (and her built-in food supply) wouldn't be home for another two hours. He himself had nothing to give to his crying baby.

It is important to follow the directions on the container carefully. Modern baby formula has been developed through years of research and study. If the formula is a powder and the instructions say to mix two tablespoons of powder with four ounces of distilled water, this is exactly how you should mix it. It's better to err by diluting the mixture too much than by using too much of the concentrate.

Bathing

Wait until the umbilical cord stump comes off before giving the baby its first full bath. This will happen in a week or two. Until then, keep this area dry. The doctor may recommend swabbing the area gently with alcohol. This keeps the site clean and helps the stub to dry. A sponge bath will do in the meantime.

Giving the baby a bath is almost an art. You'll have your hands full of a squirming, wet, slippery baby that is likely to make sudden movements. Your job is to maintain control, while doing this very gently. And with a newborn, you also have to support the head. It takes a little practice, but you'll get the hang of it quickly enough.

There will be the need to "spot-clean" constantly. Changing diapers is a good example of this. Merely changing the diaper isn't enough. If you don't keep that entire area very clean and dry (and even if you do), diaper rash can become a real problem. This is easier to prevent than to treat. There are creams, ointments, and medicated wipes that will help.

For a complete bath, again concentrate on keeping this area clean. Also give special attention to areas that tend to be less open to the air, such as the armpits. The hair should be shampooed with a gentle shampoo meant for babies. You can use this washing as a time to massage the baby's scalp. Rinse the hair thoroughly, then dry briskly with a towel, and comb or brush. Toweling the baby dry can also be done with some briskness to stimulate the skin.

The entire bath shouldn't take very long. You don't want to get your baby chilled.

General Care

There are many comprehensive books on neonatal care. It's a good idea to have at least one, especially if it also contains detailed information on handling emergencies.

Most of it is basic common sense. Keep the baby warm, but not overly warm. Some sun is good, but you need to protect your child from getting too much. Be gentle and slow when handling the baby, and never pick up a newborn without supporting the neck and head. For that matter, gently support the baby's entire body. Picking it up by just an arm can easily lead to a dislocation or even broken bone.

Spanking a newborn is both cruel and useless. If the baby is crying, there is a reason for it. Striking the baby only gives it more reason to cry.

It is common practice for the doctor to put silver nitrate drops in the baby's eyes. This prevents the spread of a number of diseases. For the first few days you may need to wipe the corners of the eyes with a clean cloth. Do this very gently.

For a while you may look down at your baby only to have it look back at you cross-eyed. This is normal, as long as it is only occasional. It's also quite normal for the young baby to use just one eye while the other "drifts." This is particularly common for a baby less than two months old, but it can continue for almost two years. You can help in two ways.

One is to vary how you place the baby for rest. One time the right side of the face can be down—the next time, the left. This gives each eye a chance to be dominant—and be exercised—in turn. The other is to play games that stimulate both eyes. Something as simple as moving your head back and forth while you make silly sounds does more than just bring a smile or giggle. It helps exercise the baby's eyes.

Perhaps most important of all is to recognize that even an infant responds to love and affection. Even if you're nervous about holding your baby, you can come to be comfortable with it and enjoy it very quickly. Don't be too surprised when you find yourself rocking your baby to sleep and regretting having to put him or her in the crib.

Warning Signs and Illnesses

The trend is toward looser, more open visiting hours in the hospital. Mom isn't sick. She is pregnant or a new mother. Consequently she is allowed visitors. Even so, careful screening of visitors is important. If the hospital doesn't do this (or can't—not all diseases can be seen), it's up to you. NO ONE who is sick should be allowed to be near the baby. Its immune system isn't intact as yet. Even a minor illness can become serious in a hurry. Some even suggest that the baby should not have any unnecessary visitors for about six weeks. (Some have even suggested that this protective period extend to three months or longer.)

Then the baby comes home. Everyone wants to see it. You want to show it off. But also show some sense. The rules are the same. Screen the visitors. Keep the number of people to a minimum for at least a month or so, and firmly forbid visitation to anyone who has any disease—even a runny nose.

Keep in mind that many airborne germs survive for some time. Taking the baby out of the room is poor protection. When you return, the germs can still be there, and still be quite active.

As soon as possible, begin to take the baby's temperature. Make a chart. This will give you practice at taking the baby's temperature and, more important, give you an idea of what is normal for *your* baby at various times of the day and under various conditions. The standard 98.6° is nothing more than an average even in adults, and it fluctuates depending on time of day, activity, stress, and a variety of other factors. The body temperature of an infant swings up and down to an even greater extent. By monitoring your baby's temperature, you'll come to know what is normal for *your* child.

Just because the baby has a temperature of 99° or so doesn't mean that he is sick. You could easily find that his temperature is a full degree above normal when actually nothing at all is wrong. A half degree means virtually nothing by itself. Get used to your baby's normal range. This can prevent a lot of panic later on—and can also alert you more accurately when something *is* wrong.

Most adults take their temperature by holding the thermometer under the tongue. This isn't practical—or safe—with a baby. Taking the temperature through the anus is more accurate, but is unpleasant for the baby and brings a risk. Keep in mind that you MUST sterilize the thermometer immediately after taking the temperature if you do it this way. And use ONLY a thermometer that is meant for anal insertion.

The classic method is to place the thermometer in the fleshy part of the armpit and then hold the baby's arm down on it. This is fast (about four minutes), easy, and safe, and won't bring on a bout of crying from the baby or the risk of anal or other infection. Also, taking a temperature this way requires that you hold the baby. You can rock your child and sing soft songs while taking the temperature. This has a calming effect.

When the temperature is taken from under the arm, add one degree to the reading you get and you'll be very close to being accurate. For example, if the thermometer gives you a reading of 99°, the baby's temperature is actually 100°, or very close to it.

As we've established, crying is normal in a baby, and is even healthy. There is always a reason the baby is crying. You may not be able to determine what that reason is all the time, but the reason is there. This part of it is not a concern. The problem comes when the crying is excessive and/or non-stop for a long period, and without any apparent cause. This could be an indication that something more serious is wrong.

Often frightening for new parents is when the child has tremors during or after crying. Tremors with crying are normal as long as they are not excessive. Usually they are short quivers and stop fairly quickly. Also, the baby is conscious, alert, and basically in control.

Convulsions, on the other hand, are a bad sign. This is especially true if they occur after the baby has been quiet. Also be watchful if there has been an injury, even something as simple as falling out of bed. If you have any doubt, get to the hospital. It's possible that nothing is wrong—or the situation could be life-threatening.

It's not only possible but probable that your baby will get sick from time to time. You can help by making sure that others who are sick are kept away. This isn't easy, and becomes more complicated when you have other children. It's one thing to keep out those who don't live in your home, but quite another to quarantine those who do. Even so, do what you can to keep the baby away from anyone who might be contagious.

This also applies to taking the baby out of the house. Grocery stores, shopping malls, and other public places are filled with sick people. Your baby's immune system makes it more susceptible than older children or adults. By avoiding these places, you reduce the number of illnesses the baby will pick up. Be particularly careful during the first months.

Despite all the precautions, illness will happen. Most of the time it will be something simple the child can throw off on his own. Other times the illness could require medication. Do not self-prescribe, even for "normal" illnesses. A fever that lasts more than forty-eight hours (and many recommend twenty-four hours) warrants a call to the doctor. A high fever always does.

The doctor may tell you to give the baby a dose of a medication such as Tylenol (in liquid form), or to cool the baby in a bath. For the first, follow the doctor's directions implicitly! It can't be stressed strongly enough that you should *never* administer any kind of medication to an infant with the doctor's specific orders and directions. For the second, remember that you are trying to cool the child, not chill it.

Emergencies

Most medical emergencies come about due to accident. Sooner or later the baby or child is going to get itself into trouble in one way or another. It might swallow something it shouldn't. It might fall down. The list of possibilities is endless.

The key is prevention. Do everything you can ahead of time to prevent these emergencies from happening. Put latches on cupboard doors. Even then, put everything that is even *possibly* poisonous or dangerous well above the reach of the child.

Want to see what a baby can get into? Get down on your hands and knees and crawl through the entire house. See the world from the baby's perspective. Let your curiosity run loose. *Everything* is new and interesting to the baby. For you, that electrical outlet is an ordinary convenience used for the TV set. For the baby, it's something to taste, and the TV is something to climb or push over.

As detailed in Chapter Four, childproof your home, preferably before the baby even comes home with you from the hospital. After you've done everything you can think of, get down on your hands and knees and go through it all again. And again. No matter how many times you do it, you're going to miss something.

Even if you catch everything, you cannot—CANNOT—totally protect your child. There are too many things that are beyond your control. Preparation is also possible for these situations.

The first and best thing you can do is to check with a local hospital or other group and find out if infant CPR classes, and any other infant and child-related classes, are offered. Then enroll and attend. You won't regret it. Remember, the time for attending such classes is *before* you need them, not after.

Learning CPR techniques isn't difficult. Nor is learning how to deal with various emergencies that might arise. For example, your baby is choking. You have a matter of a couple of minutes before permanent damage sets in, and less than ten minutes before it's too late for anyone to do anything. What do you do?

Or worse, you walk in and your baby has already turned blue. The amount of time you have to react properly is now considerably less. Hesitation can mean the difference between life and death for your baby. Doing the wrong thing is just as serious.

For example, if the baby is choking, it's almost certain that it is choking on *something*. Some swallowed object. But putting your finger blindly into the baby's mouth can do two things. First, it can push the object in deeper and make the choking situation worse. Second, there is a good chance of doing physical damage to the tender tissues of the throat.

A joke tells of someone in a panic screaming, "What's the number for 911?" Unfortunately, it happens. Even more common is forgetting your address, or the nearest cross streets. More common yet is for people to be in such a panic that the 911 operator can't get the needed information to provide emergency help.

The key is to remain calm. That's easy to say—not easy to do. Run through it in your mind. Pretend that there is a real emergency. This doesn't compare to the real thing, but imagining it can help. The same is true for others in the household. It becomes somewhat like teaching those in your house what to do in any kind of emergency.

If the baby is to be left with someone, all this is true even more. Be sure to have all the important information right by the phone. This should include a large 911 at the top, followed by your phone number, address, nearest main cross street, the name and phone number of the baby's regular doctor, the phone number (and if possible, address) of where you will be, and the name, phone number, and address of the nearest relative or guardian. Some parents take it a step further and even draw a map to the nearest hospital.

You also need to leave authorization for the baby-sitter to grant permission for needed medical procedures. Preferably this should be notarized, but just a signed note is better than nothing. It should read something like:

I [your name], am the parent of [child's name], age [child's age], and do hereby grant [baby-sitter's name] permission to au-

thorize emergency medical attention for my child on this date [date or dates]. The child's doctor's name is [name] and can be reached at [phone number].

Even with this, many procedures will not be done until you are contacted. Without it, the fear of legal problems will cause many doctors and hospitals to do nothing unless the situation is immediately life-threatening. This policy is usually more relaxed with an infant, but you still need to make it clear that the person in temporary charge of your baby has your authority to do what is needed.

This brings with it a responsibility on your part. However unlikely it is that anything will go wrong during your absence, the person you select to be in charge is quite literally being put in charge of the life of your baby. This is not a choice to be made lightly.

What Is Coming?

Your baby will be able to suckle and grip immediately. There will be the obvious reactions to the external world. These begin at birth (and before), and continue to be refined. For the first weeks the baby will squirm and wiggle. Usually between the second and third weeks, the baby will be able to lift its head. Somewhere approaching the third month, your baby will be able to turn over on its own. Not long after this, he (or she) will be crawling.

The muscles and coordination continue to develop. Crawling along begins with a few feeble attempts, but before long your baby will be scooting along at high speed. Hand-eye coordination increases, as does the sense of balance. By five or six months the baby can sit up without help. By seven or eight months most babies can hold a bottle (although help may be needed for a while).

Many new parents become worried when the neighbor's

child walks at eleven months while their own is fourteen months old and still crawling. Don't be. Those first precious steps rarely occur before the tenth month, and may not happen until the eighteenth month (which is also fairly rare).

The first words can occur almost anytime. Sounds will be made from the start. Depending on more variables than can be listed, the first word could come after a few months or not until much later. Then will become (with your coaching) short sentences. As stated earlier, baby talk can only hurt— but so can talking to the child as though it is an adult. Repetition is needed, and patience.

Before you know it, the baby that may have spent the first nights at home in a cushioned laundry basket will be yanking furiously at the bars of the crib. The baby so totally dependent on you will become a human missile heading at top speed—on knees or feet—for the nearest danger. That long wait to hear the first words could soon become trying to resist saying, "Will you please be quiet for a moment?"

Do your best to be a part of everything. Changing a diaper is unpleasant now but, strange as it may sound, can leave behind many fond memories. Losing a few hours of sleep to rock your baby back to sleep in the middle of the night can be something precious to you in the future.

What Can You Do?

You are now both a husband (or mate) and a father. These bring responsibilities—and with those responsibilities comes a lot of hard work, and even more rewards. What you make of it is entirely up to you.

The way to make the most of it is to participate. Being male, you can't become pregnant, can't carry a child in your womb, can't give birth—but you can certainly be there and be an important part of it. After the child is born, you can't breast-feed the child—but feeding is only one small part of being a parent. (Don't forget that bottle-feeding can be done just as well by the father as by the mother.)

Imagine yourself locked in a room, with the only attention being regular meals. Those meals might be gourmet delights, but you will be an unhappy person. It's the same for the baby. It craves attention and the show of love. Providing this for your child has nothing to do with gender.

You can hold your child, play with your child, sing songs to it, even tell it a story. It will be some time before the child understands the words. The love and caring behind it will be understood much, much sooner. There are also strong indications that this kind of attention increases the baby's intelligence.

Some baby talk is okay. You can goo-goo and make silly noises. This is enjoyable for both of you. Babies love to play. Just remember that the baby is learning. If the *only* thing the baby hears is baby talk, this is how the child is learning the language. All this begins fairly early, and influences the child for a lifetime.

These days both still and video cameras are fairly inexpensive. If you don't own either, consider making the investment. If you can't afford it, perhaps a friend or relative can lend you a camera on occasion. You might miss the daily activities, and probably the holidays, but at least you can get a record of your child(ren) at various ages and stages of growth. Years from now, even the ordinary daily activities will be special.

Overall, you will soon learn that raising a child is hard work. When it's a team effort between both the mother and father, the job is much easier, much more rewarding, and helps to give the child those solid basics that will carry the child through life.

14

Doctors and More Doctors

*W*elcome to the world of medicine. You're going to see a lot of it over the coming years.

During the pregnancy Mom probably saw the doctor once per month, then once per week as the due date approached. Even if delivery was handled by a midwife, it's likely that a doctor was apprised. (Many midwives have a relationship with a doctor or hospital, just in case something goes wrong.)

Your child was born and was examined, possibly by the same doctor—possibly by a specialist—possibly by another doctor you have selected for your child.

Mom will have at least one more visit to her doctor. Visits to the baby's doctors have just started. It is generally recommended that the baby be examined by a doctor once each month for at least the first six months, then at six-month intervals until the child is two, and yearly thereafter.

Then there will be the various childhood illnesses, immunizations, physicals, accidents. . . .

It's not at all unusual for a family to have at least three regular doctors—one for Mom, one for you, and one for the children. Add to this specialists who are needed from time to time, the nurses, lab technicians, etc., and you'll find that your family has quite a medical staff working for it. (And don't forget the dental exams and work that will be needed.)

Exactly how you handle it will depend on your personal preferences and on circumstances. You might prefer a pediatrician for your children, and hopefully will never have the need of a doctor who specializes in broken bones (or worse). Or it could be that your entire family will use the same general practitioner for most things.

Why Decide Now?

Whatever route you choose, the real key is to find the doctor(s) *before* the need arises, as it certainly will. The advantages of having a "regular doctor" should be obvious.

Medical help is readily available across the country. You can go into a hospital or clinic, sign the proper forms, pay the fees, and you will get help. There are many clinics, services, and programs all set up to provide health care, sometimes at no charge (sometimes even with "no questions asked"). The problem is that these situations involve strangers treating strangers.

Most of the time this doesn't matter. Any competent physician can diagnose and treat various illnesses. Giving an inoculation certainly doesn't require personal knowledge of the patient.

Because of this and other reasons, some people don't begin looking for a doctor until one is actually needed. Although this is usually not a terrible problem, it can bring complications.

A regular patient-physician relationship gives the doctor an increasing familiarity with the patient. The patient—your child in this case—becomes more than marks on a chart. Trends are more likely to be spotted. For example, does this child have recurring throat infections? Which antibiotics seem to work best? If the doctor is the same all the time, the medical records will be right there, and eventually so will the memory.

That familiarity extends to the child. Even an infant can come to recognize individuals who are seen regularly. As you probably realize yourself, visiting the doctor can be frightening. Knowing the physician can help reduce this. Especially as your child grows, he or she will be much more comfortable with a doctor the child knows.

Perhaps one of the most important reasons for selecting a regular doctor early is access. When treatment is needed, if the child has a regular doctor, all you need to do is call for an appointment. This is much more difficult to do if the doctor has never seen you before. Some doctors are so busy that they don't readily accept new patients. Most will give priority to their regular patients. You could easily find yourself having to call a number of doctors before one will accept you at all, and even then you will probably have to wait for an appointment.

Having a regular doctor doesn't cost anything. You pay for any needed services, of course, but in between there are no charges. (However, a doctor who knows you is more likely to be flexible if you are "a bit short.") Consequently, it's like making an investment in the future, but without any cost.

The Mother's Doctor

This was discussed in depth in Chapter Three. Now, unless the doctor handling the delivery was a general practitioner, this doctor will be largely out of the picture.

Ob-gyn (obstetrics gynecology) is a specialty dealing only with medical situations that affect women. This includes pregnancy and birthing, but does not extend very far into neonatal care. It's possible that this doctor will perform the circumcision on a male baby, and will certainly give the baby its first physical exam—but after that, your baby will need another doctor. This same doctor might continue to serve the mother, and might even take care of your child later on if it's a girl. Neither is of any help now for your baby.

This doctor will be an excellent source for a recommendation, however. Since neonatal care follows immediately after the birth, the ob-gyn often knows several pediatricians. The best time to select the baby's doctor is before the birth.

General Options

One option involves all the various choices of medical services such as hospitals, clinics, and so on. Even if you have decided to select a regular physician for your baby (and you should), it's wise to be as well informed as you can be about what is available.

Hopefully you will never need the services of a hospital emergency room. Still, the time to find out about the nearest one is well before the emergency arises. The same applies to other local services that might be available (including courses on CPR, first aid, lifesaving if you have a pool, etc.). Many of these services, you will never need. Others can make life easier and less expensive, and health care more complete.

In choosing a doctor, you have two basic choices—pediatrician or family physician.

The pediatrician is a specialist in treating children. This brings an obvious advantage at times. This doctor treats children and *only* children. A doctor who only rarely sees children may be perfectly competent, but could miss something the pediatrician sees automatically. There are some disadvantages, however.

The first is that specialists tend to charge more. They've gone through all of the training of a general practitioner, plus additional education in the specialty. Sometimes the difference in cost is minor. Other times the difference is substantial, especially if the doctor has knowledge and/or skills unique even within the specialty.

Second, because of the specialty, the time will come when you'll be looking for a doctor again. Most pediatricians treat children from birth to about age twelve or thirteen. Some will continue to treat through the teenage years, or at least part of those years. Sooner or later, though, the child ceases to be a child and will have to face a new doctor. While this is a long time off (considering that your baby has just been born), it's something you need to take into account.

The GP (general practitioner, also called a family doctor) is a specialist in his or her own right. That specialty is general medicine. They handle just about anything and everything that comes along, while also keeping track of the specialists who are called in when the situation is beyond the GP's range of experience or skill. Many are qualified to perform complex surgery or have some other specialty.

Some, for example, concentrate on the family and generally avoid older patients. Others are just the reverse. In your case you are looking for a doctor who is accustomed to treating children. You might consider this a "step down" from a doctor who treats *only* children, but this choice brings the advantage that the doctor will continue to be your child's primary-care physician even after your baby grows up. The familiarity will remain.

Either way, fewer and fewer doctors are in sole practice. There will usually be one or more partners. This works well for both the doctor and the patients. It allows you to have access to a doctor twenty-four hours per day, seven days per week, all year long. No one individual could provide that all alone.

With most of these partnerships, your child will see the same physician almost all of the time. A partner will usually come in only if the primary doctor is unavailable. The partners share this responsibility, filling in for each other. The doctors can then "have a life" and even take vacations, while the patients are assured of constant access to medical care.

Interviewing

As stated in Chapter Three, whichever doctor you choose, remember that the doctor is your employee. You have the right to hire or fire. You also have the right to ask questions of your prospective employee before you hire. As long as you are polite—and your questions make sense—most physicians don't mind such an interview. Many actually welcome it. The doctor may have become a doctor because of caring, but this is still a business deal—for both of you.

Before you go in for the interview, find out whether the doctor charges for this. Many do, and are justified in that the time involved is the same as if they were with a patient. Whether the doctor charges or not, do your best to keep the interview short (but take note if the doctor seems to be rushing you).

The list of questions to ask will depend on your needs.

However you feel personally, the gender of the physician is largely irrelevant. The only possible concern would be future embarrassment for your child. A little girl might not like being examined by a man, and a little boy might not like being examined by a woman. If the child has grown up with the doctor, however, this is rarely a concern.

The age of the doctor was also discussed in Chapter Three. The younger doctor may (or may not) be familiar with the latest innovations. The older doctor has more years of practical experience. The only real concern in regard to age is to generally avoid choosing a doctor who plans to retire in a year or two.

Competency is almost impossible to rate. You can contact your state's medical board to find out if there are any outstanding complaints against the doctor, but even this can be misleading. Sometimes an incompetent doctor "gets away with it" for many years. Other times a highly capable doctor gets caught up in a string of false or unjustified complaints. It helps if the doctor you are considering has been recommended by one you already trust.

For the most part, you have to make a personal judgment on your feelings after talking with the doctor. From there, experience in how this doctor handles things will tell you if it's time to find another doctor.

Even more difficult is finding out about the competency of any other partners involved in the doctor's practice. Obviously (or hopefully) the doctor feels that the partners are competent or he wouldn't be allied with them. This doesn't mean you can't ask who the partners are, how many there are, what they do, what their specialties are, and what they can offer.

Related are the doctor's hospital affiliations. As with the birth of the baby, the facilities and attitudes of the hospital can play a major role. When your baby was being born, it was important that the hospital allow—and even encourage—you to be there. Now that your baby is in the world, there is a similar concern. If your child has to be in the hospital overnight, does the hospital allow at least one of you to room in? (This assumes, of course, that there isn't a valid medical reason to separate you from your child.)

Don't be afraid to ask about standard charges. There is no way for the doctor to give you a list of every possible charge or fee, but you have the right to know what to expect to pay for a standard office visit, and for other common services such as immunizations. Most doctors allow telephone consultations (within reason) for their regular patients without additional charge. Some will charge extra.

One of the reasons you are seeking a primary-care physician for your child is to have access. It is fair to ask about making contact after normal office hours. Ideally you should have access in emergency situations at any time of the day or night. (Be a good patient, however, and be considerate.)

There are many controversies in medicine and child rearing. You will probably want a doctor who shares your own views. Some prescribe medicine almost indiscriminately, while others don't seem to believe in medications unless absolutely needed. The same might be true of various surgical procedures.

He might press for your baby boy to have a circumcision, while you don't believe in it—or might accuse you of child abuse and refuse to perform the operation, while you want your child to have it. Removing the tonsils is another area of controversy. In the past it wasn't unusual for the tonsils to be removed almost as a matter of course. Most doctors today see it as a viable option, but only after other methods of treatment have been exhausted.

Asking just these two questions will give you a good idea about how the doctor feels about resorting to surgery. The general rule of thumb is that the doctor should be willing to use surgery when needed, but not be overly enthusiastic.

Immunizations

Still another area of controversy is immunization. Virtually every public school in America requires a record of immunization before the child will be allowed to attend. Some, however, believe that immunization is potentially dangerous. (Most physicians recommend it.) This is a matter you will have to decide for yourself. The topic is well beyond the scope of this book, but you are advised to study it thoroughly and with an open mind.

In the past, many children died due to childhood illnesses. Vaccines have been developed that cause the child's body to develop an immunity. This doesn't totally remove the risk but so greatly reduces it that childhood deaths by these diseases are almost unheard-of (among immunized children).

There are seven main immunizations. These are for diphtheria, pertussis (also called whooping cough), tetanus, polio, measles, mumps, and rubella (also called German measles). You will probably hear of DTP, which is short for diphtheria, tetanus, and pertussis. This is probably the single most critical immunization. The immunization for measles and mumps is often combined, and may be referred to as MMR (for measles, mumps, and rubella). Almost nonexistent now is the vaccination for smallpox. There are also many "optional" vaccinations, most of which are not recommended for children. A few of these are typhoid, typhus, influenza, meningitis, pneumonia, and spotted fever.

Diphtheria is bacterial. The nose, throat, tonsils, and lymph nodes become infected. Treatment is difficult, and when it's contracted, the child often dies. Even those who survive may suffer heart damage due to the toxins produced by the bacteria. The vaccine, developed in the World War II era, works well. Adverse reactions to the vaccine are rare.

Tetanus affects the nervous system. It is sometimes called lockjaw because one of the common symptoms is a stiffening of the jaw. It also causes painful spasms in the voluntary muscles, sometimes leading to paralysis. It usually enters the body through a wound, which includes insect bites. Untreated, it is almost always fatal, with the patient dying from suffocation and sheer exhaustion.

Pertussis (whooping cough) is still very common. It is a highly contagious disease of the respiratory system. The name *whooping* comes from the strangling cough that so often accompanies the disease. It is fatal most often in children under the age of one, but can cause serious and sometimes permanent complications with older children. The vaccine itself is, unfortunately, not always effective.

Polio (*poliomyelitis*) affects the spinal cord. It is rarely fatal, but can lead to paralysis. Most often, however, this viral infection is mild and causes no damage. It is still rampant in some parts of the world. Immunization is simple and believed to be very safe.

Measles is caused by a virus. It is very contagious and affects the respiratory system, the eyes, and the skin. Although it is not considered dangerous in itself, it can easily lead to pneumonia, which can be fatal, and to encephalitis (an inflammation of the brain). Ear problems, including possible permanent damage, may also occur.

Mumps is also viral and contagious. One symptom is a swelling of the parotid glands, located beneath the ears. This can cause a swelling of the face in these areas, on either one or both sides. Although a very uncomfortable disease, it rarely causes difficulties. It can, however, bring on encephalitis and ear damage. In adults, mumps can cause infection and damage to the testes or ovaries, and can bring on mastitis (inflammation of the breasts). In extremely rare cases, adults may become sterile.

Rubella is also called German measles. It is similar to measles, but the symptoms tend to be much more mild. It presents no real dangers other than to a woman who is pregnant. If she contracts the disease in the first months of the pregnancy, the fetus can be severely and permanently damaged.

Immunization for diphtheria, pertussis, tetanus, and polio usually takes place at two months, four months, six months, and eighteen months, when the child is four to six years of age, and a booster at fourteen to sixteen years. Although not all agree, many physicians recommend a booster every ten years, even for adults. Immunization for measles, mumps, and rubella usually takes place at fifteen months. Many schools now require a second measles immunization.

The shots are almost painless. The child is likely to jump, and to cry for a few moments after, but this is more from surprise than from pain. When one child began to cry after a shot, the mother asked, "Oh, did one of those little beetles bite you?" The child nodded his head, and that was that.

Some immunizations are given orally. There is certainly no pain, but some children object to the taste, or resist having the ampule put into the mouth.

Programs are available on county, state, and federal levels in an effort to see that all children are immunized. A push is on to make some of these "no questions asked." The goal is to make the vaccines available to every child, whether a legal citizen or illegal alien. The idea behind this is that immunization is very inexpensive, while trying to treat a child who has contracted one of these diseases is expensive. It's also sometimes futile, which results in much suffering, and often death.

You may choose to use one of these programs or clinics, or might prefer that the child's regular doctor handle it. The doctor or clinic will provide a "shot record," which is a small card on which the immunizations are recorded. Keep this card in a safe place. Bring it along each time so it can be updated, then store it safely at home again.

Regular Exams

As previously stated, the usual recommendation is that the child be examined monthly for the first six months, then at six-month intervals until the child reaches the age of two, and yearly after that until the child is at least five. The reason is that the most risky months are the first ones. From there, as the child's body and immune system develop, the risks become increasingly less.

For many, the schedule seems to be almost irrelevant. Children will naturally contract a number of illnesses. Your child could very easily be in to see the doctor more often than the given schedule. Be aware, however, that "physical exams" are different from "diagnostic exams." The diagnostic exam is to find the cause of a particular illness, and to treat that illness. The physical exam is more complete and thorough, and performed best when the child is healthy.

Consult your physician about the schedule he or she recommends. It may match the preceding schedule, or may vary.

Emergencies

Get and study at least one high-quality first aid manual. Many of these are available, often at low cost. Become familiar with basic first aid. Also invest in a good first aid kit (and learn how to use it).

To repeat what has been said several times, take the time to attend classes. CPR classes are held by many hospitals and fire departments across the country at little or no cost. The biggest mistake many people make is to not take advantage of these courses. The second greatest is to take just one and never repeat. Going a second time refreshes your memory.

Childproofing your home is an impossible task. No matter how complete you are, your baby is certain to find ways to get into trouble. Most of the time this will involve little things. Other times it could call for a race to the hospital or a call to 911. The more potential dangers you remove, the safer your child will be. Remember—prevention is a whole lot easier than dealing with an accident.

You don't choose the emergency medical personnel as you do the family physician. Basically they are just there.

Officers with the police and fire departments have some emergency training. EMTs (emergency medical technicians) are often attached to fire departments, as are paramedics. There are also separate paramedic units, some allied directly with a hospital, others working with an ambulance service (or airlift service).

What happens at the hospital depends on many things, beginning with the level of care that hospital is set up to provide. Some provide only basic care—others can handle just about any emergency. Almost every large city has at least one hospital that specializes in problems with children.

The typical emergency room is usually fairly quiet. For the most part they handle medical problems that are fairly minor. For example, if your child is running a fever and it's 3:00 A.M., the situation is probably not life-threatening, just inconvenient. Your doctor may suggest that you go to the emergency room—not because it is an emergency but just to be safe.

The person behind the desk is often a qualified nurse, trained and capable of handling triage. This means she makes a fast determination of how serious the problem is. If it's very serious, the medical staff jumps into action. If it's not serious, you may have to consign yourself to waiting your turn.

If it is a true emergency, expect to be separated from your child. Hopefully you will be kept informed, but in an emergency situation, the situation itself is the most important thing.

Once again, you can help prevent this from ever happening by being safe in your home. The more dangers you remove, the less likely it will be that you'll ever have to worry about an emergency.

What Can You Do?

Like it or not, at least for the next few years you'll be dealing with a lot of doctors. These years in your child's life are not to be taken lightly. Illnesses that you can throw off as an adult can cause serious damage to a child. An untreated respiratory infection, for example, can very easily extend itself and cause a hearing loss.

If you look on containers of "children's" medications, you will notice that most warn you clearly that even the smallest dose should not be given to a child of less than fifty or sixty pounds or under six years without a physician's direction. Follow those warnings. But this also means that, once again, you need the services of a doctor.

Whether you choose a family practitioner or pediatrician—whether you intend to use clinics or other facilities for most of the basic care—find a doctor to provide primary care for your baby. Start your search before the baby is born if possible. In making your choice, and in staying with that doctor, always remember that you are the employer—and also that the reason you hired this person was for his or her expertise and training. You have the right, at all times, to seek another medical opinion or another doctor.

Don't be shy about asking for an interview. In fact, if the doctor refuses, it could be a bad sign. Even if the reason for refusal is as simple as "I'm too busy," that same excuse might come up again when you really need the doctor. (Be clear in your request for an interview that you will take only ten or fifteen minutes.)

Also, don't be shy to ask questions as the relationship begins and grows. It's not the job of the doctor to train you as a parent, but a part of it *is* answering your questions (within reason). You might ask for a recommendation on the brand of thermometer to buy, or what a home first aid kit should contain. He might be able to recommend reliable books on first aid, emergencies, and parenting in general.

There are many such books available. Some list the common diseases, with symptoms and methods of treatment. A few even give flow charts to help you match the symptoms with the disease that might be causing it. These can be excellent guides, but remember that they should never replace professional medical help.

Another kind of reference is one that lists medications. For most, such a reference book is of little use around the house, but libraries have them, also. Ideally the doctor will tell you about possible side effects, and the druggist will repeat the information. It doesn't always work this way, unfortunately.

The son of one young couple suffered chronic throat infections. Antibiotics would take care of one bout, but another would follow very soon. The primary-care physician referred them to a throat specialist. She looked at the medical records and told the parents very small amounts of the bacteria were surviving in the folds of the tonsils. The major part of the infection was being handled, which was why the baby seemed to get well on antibiotics, but the surviving bacteria soon bloomed again.

She didn't want to use surgery. At least not until trying a different kind of medication. She explained thoroughly and clearly what she was trying to accomplish and why. She forgot to tell them that this medication causes the urine to become a bright orange. As it was, they'd looked up this drug in a reference book and learned of the side effect. If they hadn't, they might have panicked, thinking there was blood in the urine.

Take the time to become informed, and to stay informed. The more you know, the better off you, and your child, will be.

15

The New Father

*B*eing a father isn't just a matter of having another mouth to feed. It's a whole new way of life. Having a child in the house changes everything.

In those first months, your baby will sleep a lot but will rarely sleep through the night. You can expect to be awakened every night. After a while, both you and Mom are going to feel the exhaustion. You'll soon come to understand why parents celebrate, "My baby slept through the whole night!"

Right from the start it's going to seem that there is a never-ending need for various baby supplies. Unless you use a diaper service, there will be box after box after box of diapers. Later you'll probably have so many jars of baby food, you'll start inventing ways to use the empties. (They're great for holding small nails, screws, nuts, etc.)

Clothes will be outgrown before they wear out. Even if you use disposable diapers or a service, the washing machine is likely to be used heavily. Baby will feed—baby will spit up. Baby's clothes are changed. Baby spits up again. And if you're holding baby at the time, your own clothes will also end up in the laundry room.

Everything you do, everything you try to plan, will revolve around the baby and the baby's needs. Should you want to go out to a movie or out for dinner, a baby-sitter will be needed. Spontaneity will be, for a while, a thing of the past.

Your home itself will have changed. The cupboards and cabinets will have latches to keep the baby out. For a while you'll find yourself getting frustrated because every time you try to open one, the door comes to a dead stop in your fingers. Electrical outlets will have protective plastic caps that have to be removed—and then replaced. Doorknobs may already have protective covers, which keep the child out but which aren't that easy for adults to use, either.

Mom is very likely to have changed, too, or at least will seem to have changed. Taking care of the baby is hard work. This and the nights of broken sleep will be tiring for her (and you). Time and attention she once spent on you will be divided.

As your child grows, things will get both better and worse. Typically the baby will go from the breast to the bottle to the jars of baby food to more solid food that has to be meticulously cut into tiny pieces (while your own supper gets cold). The baby will go from total dependency to crawling, then to walking. From making only noises to not seeming to know when to be quiet.

It's an absolutely wonderful time! At least it can be, if you let it. There will be frustrations, but also great fulfillment.

Much of this began during the pregnancy. You probably experienced delight and pride, but along with those emotions probably came fears and anxieties. Will you be able to handle the finances? Will the baby be healthy? Will Mom be okay? How will you be as a father?

During the pregnancy these and other questions were very real, but most were more distant. Now you are a father.

Be Involved—Stay Involved

Hopefully you've been involved throughout the pregnancy. If so, everything will be much easier. No matter how concerned you were at the beginning, those months of involvement helped to inform you, and to get you more used to the whole idea. Make a comparison.

One father has had nothing to do with anything all along. He didn't attend classes, never went to the doctor with his wife, didn't really pay any attention. A second father has done just the opposite. He has done everything possible to be a part. Then the day comes and a baby is handed to each father. The first father is going to be just as lost as he has always been. The second father may feel a little uncomfortable at first, but he will experience parenthood.

The same is true as time passes. The father who doesn't take part in his child's life leaves two holes—one in himself and one in the child. The father who gets involved and stays involved brings happiness to himself, his wife, and his children.

Even if you missed some parts of the pregnancy and the birth, it's not too late. In fact, the importance of your role has just increased. You are a father now, which is every bit as important as being a mother. The child raised in a solid home, with two parents, is happier, more successful, and less likely to get into trouble.

It may not be easy. You come home exhausted from a hard day at work and want to relax in front of the television for a while. Keep in mind that Mom will also be tired—especially so if she works outside the home. Sharing in the chores and duties is more than just the fair thing, however. It can create (or strengthen) a bond.

Parenting is a team effort. Even genetically it is a team effort. The child is half you, half her. Let this notion continue into the rearing of your child.

"I'd never held a baby before," said one new father. "I guess it's typical to feel that you're going to hurt the child. Then one evening I was rocking my new daughter while my wife was cooking dinner. She fell asleep on my shoulder. In her sleep she made little movements and little noises. I was enjoying myself so much, I didn't want to put her in the crib to eat dinner. I could have spent the whole night right there."

As the years go by, there will be many firsts. The first word, the first time the baby walks, the first solid food, going to school for the first time. . . . All these things, even changing diapers, can build memories that will last you all your life. (Don't forget to capture these moments on film and video.)

Being involved means also being involved with Mom.

This starts even before the pregnancy. As an ideal, you and Mom were a team before she became pregnant—or at least became one during the pregnancy. During the pregnancy you should have been going to classes with her, reading books, discussing the future and all the other things that build toward parenting.

Especially in that last month, she needed your help more than ever. That is an uncomfortable month, and one that is often filled with the greatest level of anxiety for her (and for you). Your support during that month, and some judicious pampering, was important.

Then came the birth itself. It is hoped that you were there for it. If you weren't, then all the support and involvement through the pregnancy probably went a long way toward helping Mom through the event.

Now that the baby is born, your importance hasn't stopped. Mom will have several weeks of recovery, followed by years of trying to raise the child. While it's possible for a single parent to handle the job, it works out so much better when the father is involved with *both* the mother and the child.

The mother's diet during the pregnancy was important. It continues to be. A balanced diet helps the recovery, makes breast-feeding easier, and encourages good health in general. There is certainly nothing wrong with bringing her a box of candy now and then—but there is also nothing wrong with you playing an important part in the meal planning, grocery shopping, cooking, and, of course, cleaning up after.

This doesn't mean you should monitor her diet like a dictator. That can be taken as an effort to control. All you really need to do is become involved in making sure the meals are balanced. Remember that a balanced diet is good for you, too.

The same applies to exercise. It was of benefit all during the pregnancy, and is essential throughout life for good health. Exercise helps any wounds to heal, and speeds recovery. In the last month of the pregnancy, and for about a month after the birth, the exercise should be mild. The doctor *may* order total bed rest for some, but this is rare. Far more often Mom will be encouraged to get some exercise, even if only by walking, as soon as she can. This can be gradually increased until she is fully recovered and has returned to normal.

Exercising alone is usually pretty boring. Having a partner makes quite a difference, and makes it easier to stick to the regimen. The encouragement you can provide is especially important right after the birth, and more so if she had a C-section. Many times even walking can be painful for a while. Mom might be hesitant to do anything, because of the pain and for fear of causing herself harm (such as ripping out the stitches).

In short, become as involved as you possibly can. If something feels awkward at first, don't worry. It will soon become routine and comfortable.

Society's "Rules"?

Early in the research for this book I interviewed a woman who told me very clearly that a man can't possibly understand what the pregnant woman goes through. Interestingly, this woman had never been pregnant herself, had never attended a birthing, had never even held a newborn in her arms. To her, although she'd had less actual personal exposure to it, I'm male, she is female, and therefore she knows all about it, and I ("You're just a male, Gene!") know nothing.

During the pregnancy, you may have felt left out, even pushed aside. This could continue after the birth. Although the attitude is changing, some still have the idea that the father has no business even trying to be a part of the pregnancy, as though his role was finished the moment he "planted the seed." More than a few books on pregnancy talk of how pregnancy is "a thoroughly feminine experience" which the male can't possibly understand (and shouldn't try). One book went so far as to offer as proof the bold statement that the average father spends just seventeen seconds per week with his children.

The statement is obviously false. Yet it reflects a general attitude that the father is less important than the mother, and that a woman, being a woman, is automatically and naturally a better parent.

As you face attitudes that say you are of secondary importance, the female often faces the attitude that she isn't a complete woman unless she wants to have children. Even if she isn't taught this directly, she is surrounded by it. Little boys are encouraged to play sports—little girls are encouraged to play with dolls. Little boys are asked early what they want to be when they grow up. Often it's merely assumed that the little girl will grow up, marry, and raise a family.

All of this is changing, if slowly. The point is that common attitudes are often nothing more than habit. Being a good parent has nothing to do with gender. If someone tells you it does make a difference . . . they're wrong. Just because you are male doesn't make you less able to parent—*wanting* to parent certainly doesn't make you less of a man.

Even this is changing in society, and for the better. As more and more fathers take their place as Dad, the prejudices against fathers begin to fade. You might find yourself receiving compliments about being such a good and caring father. Recognition of the value of the father can also be seen in advances such as having diaper-changing tables in the men's rest rooms as well as in the women's.

Confusion

Confusion is normal, both during the pregnancy and after. For many men, all this is new. A part of this goes back to societal attitudes. It's possible that you've had very little exposure to pregnancy or babies. A boy or teen who likes to baby-sit is sometimes ridiculed. For a girl it is quite common. The end result is that many men have never held a baby before, or changed a diaper, until it's with their own new child.

You will be told again and again, including in this book, that one of your most important roles during the pregnancy and birthing is to provide understanding and support for the mother. This is both correct and needed. The problem is that the advice is so often vague. Also, much about this role is unfamiliar.

All this comes at a time when you are facing your own set of worries and anxieties. All the concentration is on the mother. The fact that you might be dealing with skewed emotions yourself is largely, sometimes entirely, forgotten. You're left to cope all on your own while simultaneously being told that you need to be there for Mom, no matter what. All of a sudden you are expected to be a nurturer, when society has stressed all along that this is the role of the female, not the male. The man never put into this position before is bound to feel confused and lost.

The primary key to overcoming confusion is knowledge. The more you know, the better. Don't rely on this book alone. There are many fine books out there that cover pregnancy, birthing, and caring for the baby. Don't worry that they are aimed at the mother. It's the information that matters. Become informed.

Second, get involved. This brings its own familiarity. The more you feel a part of it, the less you feel lost. Some fathers get so involved that eventually Mom comes to Dad for information or advice.

Quite often, just talking helps (and talking is part of being involved with Mom). As you listen to her fears and worries, you might come to understand your own better. You will also get a better feel of what she needs from you. If you make this time together one of sharing, both of you will benefit.

Never allow the talks to become a competition or complaint session. That's not the purpose, and in fact, goes against the purpose. If she is complaining, try your best to listen and learn. She just may have a valid point. When expressing any complaints you might have, don't let them become personal.

Remember, too, that this shouldn't be forced. You might have it in mind that you want to sit quietly and talk. Mom might be too tired, or may want to watch a certain movie on television. This isn't difficult to understand. You've certainly had your own times when you wanted to do one thing while someone else had other ideas. Be patient.

Jealousies

Jealousies are also normal. Throughout the pregnancy and birth, the attention was on the mother. After the birth, the attention will be on the baby and mother. You can very easily feel left out and unimportant. It's not at all unusual for the new father (or the old father) to feel that his life is falling apart.

In the beginning of the pregnancy Mom might be too sick to pay you much attention. During the pregnancy her fears of harming the baby, however unfounded, can psychologically cause her to hold back. It's even possible that her mixed feelings and fear of the actual birth could cause her to show anger toward you. Add to this the change in her hormones.

It's easy to come to feel that you've lost control of everything. That you have been shoved into last place. And once the baby has been born, everything can seem to be amplified. If you want to do something, go somewhere, spend some time with your wife—the baby always has to come first. Your own needs and wants come later.

In interviews, the feelings of jealousy showed in both directions. Most often it was the father who admitted to feeling a little jealous and left out—and then feeling guilty because of it. But this is not just a gender-related thing. Several mothers spoke of how the husband was so dedicated to the baby that *she* felt ignored.

One spoke of how her husband would come home from work, rush past her and head straight for the baby. If the child was awake, he barely had a word for her. If the child was asleep, the constant topic of conversation was the baby. Before the birth he would sometimes bring her small romantic gifts. Now he came home only with things for the baby.

"I must be a terrible mother," she said, "to feel jealous of my own baby."

It's mere human nature.

There is also the possibility that Mom will show signs of jealousy toward you. Even when you are very involved with the raising of your child, chances are good that a larger portion of the responsibility falls to her. This can make it seem that you have freedoms she has lost (which is very possibly true).

The best cure for jealousies is to make it a point to spend some time together, just the two of you. It doesn't have to be often. Once in a while is enough. Be aware and prepared for even the best plans to go astray, however. You might have planned to go out for dinner and dancing on a Saturday, made the reservations, hired a baby-sitter, gassed and washed the car, even bought flowers to make the evening more romantic. Then Saturday afternoon the baby gets sick. Or the baby-sitter cancels. Maybe the car refuses to start. There might even be a huge storm that sweeps through town, knocking out power or making travel impossible.

Don't let it stop you. If Saturday doesn't work out, try for Sunday, or the following Wednesday. If all you can squeeze in is a few hours, fine. A whole weekend away might be too much for either of you, especially with a newborn.

Don't forget the possibilities right there at home. Newborns can drive you crazy by not sleeping through the night. The mixed blessing is that there are hours when the child *is* asleep and both of you have some energy left. Much of the time this will be spent in catching up on normal chores that have been missed because of caring for the baby. At times, however, let those chores wait for an hour. Use that hour for yourselves.

It doesn't have to be anything fancy. Watching TV together can be very satisfying. If the baby is asleep at dinner, make it a point to help with the cooking—or cook for the two of you while Mom rocks the baby to sleep (or vice versa). There are many simple ways of spending time together, or making the time.

If Mom seems to always be too busy, with every spare moment spent cleaning the house or doing other things, consider that this might be a sign that you are not helping enough. By chipping in more, you get more involved, reduce your jealousies—and hers. Meanwhile, you help to create the time both of you need.

Siblings

One of the problems many parents face is in bringing home a new baby when another child is already there. Imagine a three-year-old child who has been the center of attention for all of his or her life, and is then suddenly thrust into the background. Even to a child it's obvious that the cause of the lack of attention is that new baby.

You've been pushed aside. So have the other children. And just as it is natural and necessary for the baby to take precedence over you, it is the same concerning the other children. The difference is that the sibling child may not be mature enough to handle the situation.

The sibling rivalry can easily become more important in the future. The children grow and develop. They become individuals who are more and more aware. It's not unusual for them to compete with one another. You might find yourself breaking up fights between them. At times it will seem that no matter what you do, the kids will be jealous of one another. Susan got new shoes—and Betsy is jealous, somehow forgetting that she got new shoes just two weeks before.

Remember to treat each child as an individual, and according to age and abilities. It's unfair, and usually illegal, to leave a five-year-old in charge of a one-year-old. It's equally unfair to expect that five-year-old to *not* be a child, and to understand the logical explanation of why he can't have that new tricycle because the baby needs a crib—or why his birthday party has to be canceled because the baby is sick.

Once again, right from the start, your role as parent becomes crucial. The children you already have need reassurance. There will be times when Mom can't provide it—and there will be times when *you* can't. As a team, however, it can work quite well. Perhaps you can play a game with the other children while Mom is with the baby.

Especially with older children, try to find a balance. If you *always* play with the children while Mom *always* is with the baby—or if you *always* play with Billy while Mom *always* plays with Rachel—instead of helping the child, you might be causing that child to wonder why the other parent doesn't like him or her.

Resuming Sex

It's not unusual for both of you to feel reluctant to have sexual relations at least sometime during the pregnancy. It could start very early, if Mom feels too ill to have any interest. It might wait until the last month when one or both of you fear harming the baby. During the pregnancy Mom might be almost totally unresponsive or could seem almost insatiable. The same may be true for you.

Regardless, after the birth there will be a period during which intercourse is highly inadvisable and is possibly dangerous. Depending on your habits and personalities, this may or may not be a problem. (Normally it is not unless you make it one.)

The general rule of thumb is that you should not resume intercourse until the doctor has examined Mom and has determined that she is fully healed. Most doctors recommend that you not give her *any* kind of stimulation in the vaginal area during this period. (Obviously your own body is not affected medically, but your wife may feel reluctant until the lovemaking is mutual.)

Even after she has recovered, there may be hesitation to resume sexual relations. That hesitation is more likely to be hers, but could be your own hesitation as well. Both are normal, and mostly just require patience. In a few cases, professional help may be required.

Regardless, don't be in a hurry. Applying pressure rarely does any good, and usually makes the situation worse. What would have been merely temporary if handled with patience can be nearly, or completely, permanent if pushed.

The doctor will probably recommend that you use contraception once you have begun to have intercourse again. Usually she is less fertile after giving birth. Usually the woman who is breast-feeding is also less fertile. Those who have taken this as an absolute, however, have sometimes found themselves facing another pregnancy just a few months after the last child was born. Even if the two of you are anxious to build a family, with children close in age, the general recommendation is to be sure that her body has fully recovered from one pregnancy before she enters into another. As has been stated before, "Nine months in, nine months out" is often the recommendation.

What Can You Do?

The best thing you can do is to get involved. The more involved you become, the fewer problems you'll have, now *and* in the future.

There has been a lot of attention paid to mother/child bonding. Very little of this attention concerns the bonding between the father and the child. Perhaps one reason is that it is too commonly assumed that Dad doesn't care to be as involved as the mother *has* to be. (Not enough time, upbringing, he can't breast-feed—there are plenty of excuses given, few of which are valid.)

The more you get involved, the more you can appreciate the new life that has so disrupted your own. Not only will you be better able to understand it when Mom seems to be ignoring you, you might find yourself doing the same.

Being a parent is hard work. Changing a diaper isn't

pleasant. There will be many sacrifices to make. Your life will never be the same again.

How you handle this is up to you. That extra work needed can mean less time to do things you'd rather be doing—or can be more time for doing things you've come to enjoy even more. Those sacrifices can be seen as things you have to give up—or can be seen as ways in which you expand your spirit, and ways in which you show your love.

This can be the greatest time of your life. All you have to do is let it be.

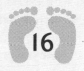

16

To Mom

*T*his final chapter is for you, Mom.

The basic theme of this book is "For every mother there is a father—for every pregnant woman there is a 'pregnant' man." The first is obvious. The second is more true than you might realize.

Pregnancy and birth is a time when the father's inability to understand what you are going through hits a peak—or seems to. He can try, but the simple fact is that *he* will never be pregnant, and *he* will never give birth, or breast-feed the baby, or go through many of the things that you will. His anatomy is all wrong for it.

What is often forgotten, especially at this time, is that just as Dad can't fully understand what Mom is going through, Mom can't fully understand what Dad is going through.

Each gender goes through unique experiences that the other gender can't completely understand. Parenthood is one of these. It's the same experience, but perceived differently by each partner (and each person—not even two women will experience or interpret it in the same way). This is due to both anatomy and upbringing.

Even so, there are more similarities than there are differences.

You're going (or have gone, or will go) through a lot. Just as you don't want Dad to forget that, don't forget that *Dad* is going through a lot, too. In some cases less than you are, in some cases more.

Especially when you're pregnant, it's sometimes difficult to believe, accept, or remember this, or that the pregnancy, the birth, and the raising of the baby can be hard on him.

What *Is* Dad Going Through?

Some fathers experience couvade syndrome. It affects at least 20 percent of them. The exact number is unknown because although this syndrome has been written about for some four hundred years, to date no serious studies have ever been done. Little is known about it, or the causes. Some claim that it's just another example of the man trying to grab attention for himself, but what the father faces, and suffers, is very real. More than a few fathers have such serious discomfort that they end up visiting the doctor. (This is a good idea. Those symptoms could indicate that something else is wrong.)

While it's fairly common for the father to experience mild and varied "symptoms," it's also true that the father will almost never feel pain or discomfort that even comes close to what Mom is, and will be, going through.

But whether he goes through this or not, he is not really pregnant. This can lead you to believe that the pregnancy doesn't really affect him. It does, even if it doesn't show.

Keep in mind that many men are raised to guard, if not

hide, their emotions. "A real man doesn't cry" is a silly attitude but is still common. Even if your husband is one who
does feel secure enough to show emotion, he was still raised
around the attitude that it's not quite right. If he didn't get
it from home, he got it from his peers.

Through the pregnancy and birthing, he will be told over
and over that he is to be supportive and understanding. (The
advice has been repeated in this book.) This is as it should
be, but it brings with it the implication that he is to swallow
whatever happens in silence, and to not burden you with his
own fears and anxieties.

You might expect him to keep his emotions and feelings
bottled up inside—which doesn't mean that they don't exist.

Now add on top of this his general lack of knowledge. He
probably got some basic anatomy classes in school, just as
you did. But he may have been shuttled out of the room
whenever the subjects of birth or babies were raised. Chances
are pretty fair that the first time he'll hold a baby or change
a diaper will be with his own child. He hasn't even played
with a doll for practice. It's all new to him—new with a living
being, his baby, and one dependent on him.

You've heard it before. "I might break it." Only rarely is
that an excuse to escape the responsibility. More often it's
brought on by plain ol' fear. And more often than you might
think, he actually feels that way—that he'll inadvertently
injure the child.

The pregnancy itself is often confusing for him. The birthing will be even more so. One woman interviewed said that
her husband was present for the birth of each of their three
children—and each time passed out on the floor. A true story
early in this book told of a father who stayed conscious, but
who took one look at his newborn child and bolted from the
hospital screaming. (He thought it was deformed.)

It's not unusual for you to have fears, especially if this is
your first child. Every twinge can bring on panic and the
lack of twinges can do the same. Will you be okay? Will the

baby be okay? Will delivery be more painful than you can bear? What if there are complications and surgery is needed?

All these fears are reasonable and normal. Believe it or not, Dad is very likely experiencing exactly the same fears—and he probably feels even less in control of them than you do. It's true that he won't be the one going through the actual delivery, but in some ways this makes it only that much worse. There is a difference between facing something yourself, and having to watch helplessly as a loved one goes through it.

Your body is going through many changes during the pregnancy. The change in the level of your hormones can cause you to do and say things. It's not unusual for a pregnant woman to occasionally feel out of control. This can be confusing for you. It is certainly confusing for the father.

The "American dream" is that the man goes out and gets the bread, while the woman raises the children. These days it's fairly common for the couple to have no choice but to both go to work, just to make ends meet, and many women want to work and feel it's important to them. Although we're growing more comfortable with the reality of the situation, many men still feel guilty if they can't earn sufficient money on their own, and have to rely on the wife to help.

Now along comes a new mouth to feed. You and Dad will owe $2,500 to the doctor and $2,500 to the hospital (more if there are complications). Then there are all the baby supplies you'll need: $350 for a crib, $20 per box for a seemingly endless stream of diapers. Visits to the pediatrician are $60 a crack. Shots, unexpected illnesses, toys, clothes, formula, baby food . . .

It's expensive to raise a child. It's also frightening! And chances are very good that it's more frightening for Dad than it is for you. More than a few fathers develop ulcers worrying about it. Or they'll start losing sleep. Or they'll become grouchy and somewhat distant.

Yes, the father faces all the fears and anxieties you do,

and a few more. He faces them in a different way, perhaps, but he does face them. Just as you need his support and understanding, he needs *yours*.

During the pregnancy most of the attention falls on you. The father is largely ignored. After the baby is born, he is pushed even further aside. This may or may not affect him. Some don't mind at all. Others come to feel very alienated. All you need do is imagine yourself being suddenly thrown into last place.

But you can help.

Getting Dad Involved

Many women have a legitimate complaint that the father doesn't play enough of a part. Forgotten is that he is often pushed out, and has been all his life. It's not easy for him to overcome all of that. He's unlikely to without your help and encouragement.

There are a number of reasons for getting Dad as involved as possible. Perhaps most important to you is how much easier it makes things—during the pregnancy, during the birth, and afterward once the new baby is home again. It also makes things easier on Dad and on the baby. The more he is involved, the better everything goes for everyone, both now and in the future.

Getting him involved begins with letting him know it's okay. It could be that he feels intimidated, or lost. It could be that he feels he's not supposed to be there. It could be that the anxieties of having to raise a family get in his way. (It could also be that he feels that he has better things to do, or that it isn't "manly" to be a real part of things.)

Pay attention to how others treat him concerning the pregnancy, birthing, and baby. He may be ignored, or even ridiculed, in ways you wouldn't see if you weren't being purposely aware. Of the men interviewed for this book, quite a few reported being made to feel unimportant, even if unintentionally.

Just as he needs to be understanding, so do you. It may take a while, but be patient, just as you would expect him to be patient. On the other hand, it's possible that a father who seems to be reluctant will suddenly throw himself into fatherhood.

The effort to get him involved, and keep him involved, is well worth it.

Sexual Relations

This may or may not be a concern. (Usually it's not.)

Early in the pregnancy, morning sickness may ruin your mood. The change in hormones can also change how you feel. For some, the desire for sex fades or even disappears. For others it increases. This may go on through the entire pregnancy, sometimes with wild swings in your emotions from one day to the next.

During the last month, having sex can cause you to fear that you might be harming the baby. It can also be very uncomfortable. (Both are also true for him.) Following the birth, the doctor will almost certainly advise that you have no intercourse, and little or no vaginal stimulation, for at least six weeks.

Even after recovery, you now have a child in your lives. The new baby has the remarkable ability to demand—and get—the center of attention. Both of you are likely to be tired. When you finally find some moments to be alone together, that time could be interrupted by a wailing baby.

How you handle this depends on your circumstances, and how you and he feel personally. No two cases are exactly alike. There is no set advice that works for everyone, all the time. It becomes a decision you have to make for yourselves.

No one should ever feel forced—male or female. (It's

nearly as common for the woman to feel the need, with the man being reluctant.) Neither should either be deprived. This doesn't necessarily mean sex. Sometimes it simply means finding the time—or making it—to just be together. It can mean simply providing the reassurance of love and caring.

What Can *You* Do?

It's obvious that you need and deserve special attention during the pregnancy, during the birth, and *at least* for the six weeks after the birth. Especially afterward, you'll need all the help you can get from Dad—and hopefully he will give it. (He might even surprise you.)

Those needs are expressed in this book, and in virtually every other book on pregnancy and birth you'll ever find. It might not seem like it at times, but Dad *does* know. Those around him aren't going to let him forget, either. Unfortunately, it's often dropped on him with the attitude "*You* made her pregnant, it's *your* responsibility."

Other than in cases of rape, pregnancy is not one-sided. It takes both to make the decision to have intercourse. Both also share in the responsibility of the results, planned or not. Pregnancy and birthing go far more smoothly when the couple work as a team. Raising the child certainly goes better.

What people often forget is that Dad has new special needs, too. He's about to become responsible for another life, same as you. He has fears and anxieties, same as you. Gender, race, hair color, etc., are all irrelevant. We are all people.

Getting married and being responsible for supporting a wife was spooky enough. Whether he shows it or not, the chances are very good that the idea of being also responsible for a baby is scaring the hell out of him. Probably, so is the idea of attending the birth.

You're going to go through mood swings, due to both psychological reasons and your hormones creating emotional havoc in your body. At times you won't be able to control yourself, and that's understandable.

Dad will also be going through mood swings, though his hormonal levels aren't shifting as they are in your own body.

Encourage him to come to the exams with the doctor. If you're too shy for the more intimate exams, at least encourage him through the middle months. With rare exception, the only thing exposed is your tummy. The first time he hears the heartbeat of the baby inside—*his* baby as much as yours—his entire attitude is likely to change.

Mostly, be a team. This is a partnership. Include him whenever you can. Defend him if someone else is trying to squeeze him out. Let him know that he is more than just a paycheck. Yes, you deserve most of the attention, but see to it that he is not left out.

Appendix:
Massage

*D*uring the pregnancy, birthing, and recovery—any time at all, actually—massage can be therapeutic in many ways. It can relieve many of the less pleasant symptoms, and just plain feels good. It's also time together. It's a time for deciding on the baby's name, for talking about your plans for the future, or for just silently enjoying each other's company.

Sometimes all she needs is a foot and leg massage. One father interviewed told of how he and his wife spent each evening sitting by the fire. She would sit on the couch in a robe, with her legs on his. Some evenings he would give her a full massage. Most evenings they shared the time together as he rubbed her feet and legs.

You don't have to be an expert with years of training, nor do you need any special equipment. All you need are your own two hands and a cushioned surface. If you wish, you can add body lotion or scented oils. Soothing background music is a big plus. (The key word here is *soothing*. Even if you prefer it normally, this is not the time for fast, energizing music.) So is subdued lighting.

Overall, there are few hard-and-fast rules. Actually there are only two.

The first is that massage should *never* cause pain. If it does, you are pressing too hard or something else is wrong. Depending on what hurts, it might be time to contact the doctor. Her abdomen, for example, might get a little tender toward the end—and you should never press hard—but the area shouldn't be so sensitive that it causes her pain. If it does, the doctor needs to be notified. Both before and after, the breasts are likely to be sensitive. This is normal. But if her breasts cause her pain even from a light touch, she might have mastitis, and again the doctor should be notified.

The second rule is somewhat similar. Don't do anything if you are in doubt. A good example of this is massaging the feet and lower legs. Done properly, this can relieve the swelling so many women suffer. However, if the edema is severe, attempting to "treat it" by massage alone can be dangerous. Treatment for severe edema requires a doctor's care.

The Basics

As just stated, the place used for the massage should be quiet, subdued, peaceful, and undisturbed. The primary goal of massage is relaxation. Soft music and dimmed lights help, but don't forget to unplug the phone. If you have other children, put them to bed first; and even then consider locking the door.

The temperature must be comfortable—not too cold, not too warm. The temperature should be seventy-five or above. Consider using some extra towels as blankets to keep her warm. These are better than using a blanket because they are easier to move and rearrange. For some, the towels make the person feel more secure.

Massage is best accomplished when the person is wearing no clothing. A back rub through a thick shirt isn't nearly as effective. Even a bra gets in the way. For some, lying nude even with a loved one is uncomfortable. (Even people married a long time are sometimes shy.) Using the towel as a drape allows her to be nude while still being covered. Just how you handle this depends on your situation.

One of the best times to give a massage is immediately after a shower or bath. In fact, this is a good place to begin. The bathing itself is relaxing. It also leaves the skin clean and more pliable. And having someone else wash you from head to foot is wonderful pampering. The closeness continues into and through the massage from there.

Be sure that she is thoroughly dry. You don't want her to become chilled. Once again this gives you a chance to add to the experience. Dry her yourself. Then, after she lies down, use a second dry towel to rub her briskly. This completes the drying and stimulates the skin. (It's also a great way to end a massage.)

The surface used should be soft and comfortable. You can buy or build a massage table if you wish. A bed, couch, or even a well-padded floor will do. They don't work quite as well as a massage table, but are adequate. (A water bed is generally not suitable. The person receiving the massage shouldn't be bounced around, as usually happens when she is lying down and you are crawling around.) One of the most important considerations is access. Ideally the person getting the massage should move very little—no more than just turning over. Ideally the person *giving* the massage should be standing and comfortable, and not have to bend over or reach.

Pillows can be used to prop various body parts so Mom is more comfortable. Toward the end, no matter how many pillows you use, she may be able to lie only on her back or side. If she has to lie on her side, most find it more comfortable with a pillow between the knees.

The massage itself can last almost any length of time. As a general rule of thumb, less than twenty minutes is too short—more than an hour is too long. The pace should be slow and relaxed. Don't force it. Don't rush it. Instead, try to develop a rhythm.

Another important factor that many forget is to maintain contact. There will be a few times when you have to break that contact, but for the most part, one or both of your hands should be touching her at all times. For example, if more lotion is needed, try to keep one hand in contact and in motion while the other hand gets the bottle. (Please note—any oil or lotion should be warmed first! If you haven't done this, forget the "constant contact" rule and warm it between your hands first.)

Your hands should also be in constant motion. Never concentrate on just one spot for a long time. Even if the massage you are giving is just for the feet and calves, rub the feet, then ankles, then calves, then back to the feet, ankles, calves. Keep moving, but in a calm, relaxed manner. Don't be in a hurry—just don't continue massaging a single area for more than about a minute.

The person receiving the massage should move very little. When you massage the arm or work on a joint, *you* do the moving. If your partner tenses or tries to help, remind her to relax. It might help if you say this and then move that limb until you and only you are moving it. It can also help if you support the limb well. This adds a sense of security. And when finished with that limb, lower it gently. *Never* just drop it.

The Three Basic Strokes

Every massage should begin and end with long, light touches. This is called *effleurage*. Your goal is not to apply any pressure. Instead, you are trying to get her skin and muscle tissues to warm up. That hot shower will help to relax the muscles. Effleurage completes this. It also brings the person "back out." At the beginning, begin light but increase the pressure slowly and gradually. At the end, decrease the pressure until you are once again using the long, gentle strokes.

If you wish, you can begin and end by using just your fingertips. More classically, the entire palm is used. The latter tends to work a little better if you are using oil or lotion. This provides a slickness and your hands can slide more easily.

Petrissage and *kneading* are much deeper. With both, always keep in mind that you are trying to help her relax. You are not trying to cause pain, nor to demonstrate how strong your hands are. You are trying for a deep massage, not a painful one.

Petrissage uses circular motions, often with the heel of the palm applying pressure. If you pay attention, you can often feel any tight muscles and will know where the greatest attention is needed. The smooth, flowing motion helps to accomplish this.

Kneading is more a combination of the palm and fingers. You will press and squeeze. It is *not* pinching, but sometimes seems to come close. As with petrissage, you are trying to find the tight muscles and work with them to help them relax.

A truly effective massage combines all three. It will begin and end with a lighter touch, but the long motions across entire areas can and should be mixed with the deeper petrissage and kneading. It might help if you think of it as smoothing an area, then digging in deeper, then smoothing it again at the end.

Feet and Legs—Hands and Arms

Edema is a common problem, especially in the ankles and legs. Fluids build up due to water retention and changes in the circulatory system. This causes a swelling. The feet and legs can also become sore simply because of the increase in weight and the change in the center of balance. In all, massaging her feet and legs during the pregnancy is one of the things mentioned again and again by pregnant women as being one of the most appreciated things.

Be careful to not tickle her feet. Few people enjoy this, and even then it does the opposite of what you are trying to accomplish. Instead, keep the pressure firm, with your hands mostly flat. Work from the toes (gently!) and up across the foot. Squeeze in from the sides (gently). Rotate the foot on the ankle, then work the ankle. Continue moving upward on the leg. In a sense, you are trying to push the trapped fluids back toward the main part of the body.

Edema can also affect the hands and arms. In any case, massage here is very similar to that of the feet and legs. A massage of the hands can be deliciously relaxing if done correctly, but remember to never squeeze or press too hard. Gently work each finger, then the hand. Rotate and work the wrist. Continue the massage up the arm to the shoulder.

The Back

A back rub feels good anytime. Late in pregnancy and often during labor, it provides relief in a way nothing else can.

Many people prefer to begin even a full massage with the back. It's a large area, in the middle of the body. Massage here helps the person relax all over so that massage of the limbs is more effective. Remember, however, that if you begin with the back, always massage the limbs toward the body.

The muscles of the back are generally broad and flat. A fair amount of pressure can be applied. Usually this works best moving toward the shoulders, but massaging toward the waist is also fine. Begin with long strokes. Even if you are not using oil or lotion, think of these first motions as spreading it across the back. Gradually increase the pressure. Then begin combining the techniques.

Be more gentle along the sides. Don't dig in. Instead concentrate more on longer, flat-handed pushes and pulls. At the shoulders, use one hand to pull the shoulder back. This relieves tension on the large muscles of the upper back, while also relaxing the joint. The other hand can be used at this time to massage that muscle.

The tissues along the sides aren't as thick. You don't need to use any deep kneading. A more shallow technique does better. Long, smooth strokes also feel good. You can vary the direction, sometimes moving upward along both sides, sometimes moving at an angle from the lower sides to between the shoulders, sometimes pulling upward along just one side toward the center of the back.

The lower back is always important, but is more so during pregnancy and labor. During pregnancy the increasing weight and changes in balance can give her a nagging backache. Later, the position of the baby can cause it to press against her. During labor, this pressure and the straining to give birth can be painful.

Massage of the lower back can be fairly deep. It will extend from the lower ribs to the top of the buttocks. Often a concentration at the base of the spine, where the buttocks separate, is appreciated. Fingers, thumbs, and palm heels are all effective. As you massage the lower back, occasionally move upward across the back again.

Some consider the buttocks the lowest part of the back rub; others think of it as the upper part of a leg rub. Actually the area is a little of both. This deep, thick muscle is often ignored due to possible sexual overtones. If Mom is comfortable with it (and you are), don't neglect it. The muscles of the back and legs both join the area.

Special mention needs to be made concerning back rubs during labor. It's possible that Mom won't want you to touch her at all. Pay attention to what she says. Also be listening to her if you are massaging. Sometimes the spots to rub at this time are different from what you would normally massage. This varies, depending on what is causing the pain. The same is true of how deep and hard you press.

The Front

After she turns over, much of the massage merely completes what you've already started. You've already massaged the backs of the legs, and perhaps all of the arms. (Some leave the arms until the person turns over.) Now you will massage the front. The basic rule is the same. Massage toward the heart.

A mistake many make is to pass over the knee as though it is merely something that divides the lower leg from the upper. It does, but is also an important joint, especially if you're carrying around an extra twenty-plus pounds. Some extra time spent on the knee can do wonders. Be aware, however, that the area might be sensitive. Pay close attention to her reactions.

How you massage the abdomen depends largely on the phase of the pregnancy and birthing. Late in the pregnancy, for example, any kind of pressure is inappropriate. A very gentle rubbing can be pleasurable, for both of you, however. Early in the pregnancy you can press harder, but it's very possible that she will be psychologically sensitive. After the birth, a somewhat deeper (but still gentle) massage of this area might feel very good to her.

As with the buttocks, there may be a reluctance to massage the breasts. Massaging the breasts is not necessarily sexual. The pectoral muscles of the upper chest sometimes get a little sore as the breasts become larger due to the pregnancy and nursing. This is one of the reasons many doctors advise the woman to wear a support bra. It reduces the strain on the supporting tissues.

As with the abdomen, exactly what you do depends on circumstances. Her breasts may become painfully sensitive at times. This is common early in the pregnancy and during nursing. The breasts could become so sensitive that even light touching is irritating.

The pectorals are like flat plates of muscle. They are massaged both individually and together. If the breasts aren't too sensitive, you can gently lift up on a breast to relieve tension on the muscle and use the other hand to massage that area.

Glossary

ABO incompatibility: A blood mismatch when the mother's blood is type O and the baby is either type A or B. Generally not serious.

Abortion: Spontaneous or induced expulsion of the embryo or fetus, generally prior to the sixth month. Miscarriage is also abortion, despite common use of the term of induced abortion only.

Abruptio placentae: Detachment of the placenta before the birth of the child. Also called "placental abruption."

Acidosis: A condition of excessive acidity (or lack of base) in the body. Generally metabolic.

ACOG: American College of Obstetricians and Gynecologists.

Afterbirth: The placenta and related membranes; or the process of these coming out.

Alpha-fetoprotein (AFP): Produced by fetus. Measuring the

level of AFP in Mom's blood can help detect a birth defect called neural tube defect (if level is high) and also Down's syndrome (if level is low).

Amenorrhea: The ceasing of the menstrual cycle, such as when a woman becomes pregnant.

Amnesic: A drug used to "block" pain by causing the patient to forget that it happened. The most common example is scopolamine. When the woman is "knocked out" for a birth, amnesics are usually used. She feels all the pain, but forgets about it afterward. Also called *amnesiac.*

Amniocentesis: Drawing off a small amount of the amniotic fluid for testing, such as for hereditary problems.

Amnion: The two inside layers of the amniotic sac (bag of waters). Sometimes used to describe the entire sac.

Amniotic fluid: The fluid in the amniotic sac. It surrounds the fetus, protecting it.

Amniotic sac: The bag of waters that surround and encase the fetus.

Amniotomy: Breaking of the amniotic sac artificially (i.e., the doctor cuts it) when it doesn't break on its own.

Analgesic: One type of anesthesia, effective in blocking nerve endings. The most commonly used analgesic for birthing is Demerol, the proprietary name for meperidine. Can also be a local anesthetic, such as lidocaine.

Anemia: A blood condition of too few red blood cells and/or too little hemoglobin and/or too little iron.

Anesthetic: Any number of drugs that reduce or eliminate sensations, particularly pain.

Anoxia: Lack of oxygen.

Antepartum: The period between conception and birth. Also called the *antenatal,* literally "before birth," period, although technically antepartum is before labor begins.

Apgar test: A method of scoring the condition of a new born baby, named after Virginia Apgar. Rated at one minute and then five minutes are heart rate, respiration, muscle tone, response to stimulation, and skin color.

Apnea: Temporary cessation of breath.

Areola: The colored area around the nipple, which enlarges and darkens during pregnancy.

Aspiration: Sucking in.

Back labor: When the uterine contractions are felt heaviest at the back; caused by a posterior presentation.

Bag of waters: Amniotic sac.

Ballottement: Examining a fetus by palpation of (pressing on to feel) the abdomen. Soft touching.

Betadine: Proprietary name for povidone-iodine. An antiseptic.

Bilirubin: An orangish pigment of bile which in turn causes a yellow tint to the skin of many newborns. A byproduct as the excess blood in the infant's body breaks down.

Birth canal: The vagina. The canal through which the baby passes during a vaginal birth.

Blood pressure: A measure of the pulse of blood. Consists of two parts, systolic and diastolic, with systolic being the height of the pulse and diastolic being the relaxed arterial pressure. A range of 100 to 140 systolic and 60 to 90 diastolic is considered normal. Often abbreviated BP.

Blood types: O, A, B, and AB, with Rh factors of positive or negative.

Bloody show: When the mucous plug from the cervix passes out of the vagina just before birth. Sometimes called just *show*.

Bonding: Attachment between the parents and the newborn.

BP: Abbreviation for blood pressure.

Bradycardia: An overly slow heart rate, signaling fetal distressor heart anomalies.

Braxton Hicks contractions: Sometimes called false labor, or more rarely, prelabor. Consists of small and usually irregular uterine contractions. Can occur any time after the third month of pregnancy. These are generally painless, and will usually go away if the mother moves or changes position.

Breast pump: A manual or electric device used to draw milk from the mother's breasts. Used to relieve engorgement, to stimulate milk production, or just to draw out the milk for use later. (If Mom wants to go shopping, Dad has something to give the baby.)

Breech: Feet-down, or buttocks-down, position of baby during birth. A complete breech has the infant sitting with its legs crossed. A frank breech has the legs straightened and up along the infant's body. A footling breech has one or both of the infant's feet down below the buttocks.

Candida: A yeastlike fungus. Formerly called Monilia.

Caput: The head.

Catching: "Catching the baby." Physically holding and removing the baby as it is born.

Caudal block: Regional anesthesia, given in the lower spine.

Caul: The membranes that encase the baby.

CBC: A complete blood test and count to determine anemia and other blood-related problems.

Centimeter: Unit of metric measurement. Equivalent to a little less than one-half inch (.394). Used to measure cervical dilation, with ten centimeters (about four inches) being 100 percent.

Cervical incompetence: Premature effacement and dilation of the cervix, the cause of about 25 percent of all miscarriages.

Cervix: The neck of, or opening to, the uterus. More correctly called cervix uteri, or "neck of the uterus."

Cesarean: Surgical removal of the baby through an abdominal incision. Often considered an emergency-type procedure. Also called *cesarean section* or, more simply, *C-section.* (Also spelled *caesarean* and *cesarian.*)

Chorion: The outer two layers (membranes) of the amniotic sac.

Chorionic villi sampling: A test to detect chromosomal abnormalities. A thin tube is moved through the cervix to get a sample of the placenta.

CPD: Cephalopelvic disproportion. A condition in which the fetal head is too large to pass through the mother's pelvis.

Circumcision: A surgical procedure to cut the foreskin on the penis.

Cleansing breath: A part of the Lamaze method. A deep breath at the beginning and end of each contraction, theoretically to provide mother and child with sufficient oxygen.

Clitoris: The center of sexual sensation for the female. Somewhat akin to the male's penis.

C.N.M.: Certified nurse midwife. A professional who is a registered nurse who also has special training from an accredited school for nurse-midwives.

Colostrum: "Early milk." A yellowish breast secretion very high in protein and calories. May occur in late pregnancy, and continues for two to three days after the birth and just before true lactation begins.

Complete: Term used to signal that the cervix is 100 percent dilated and effaced.

Contraction: In birthing, a tightening (hopefully coordinated, and usually involuntary) of the uterine muscles. Early contractions cause the cervix to dilate and efface; later contractions push baby out of the uterus and down the birth canal.

Cord prolapse: When the umbilical cord drops down through the birth canal before the baby does. An emergency situation, almost always requiring cesarean section.

Couvade syndrome: When the father feels and/or exhibits symptoms of being pregnant or in labor.

Crowning: When the top of the baby's head first peeks out of the vagina and/or causes the perineum to bulge.

CSF: Cerebrospinal fluid. Fluid from the brain and spinal cord. For testing for neurological problems, a small amount is taken by needle. Headaches the mother experiences after a spinal anesthetic has been administered may result from leakage of CSF.

Cyanosis: A lack of oxygen, causing the skin to appear blue.

Cystic fibrosis: A serious lung-damaging disease. One of the first signs is sometimes a saltiness on the skin.

Cystitis: Infection and inflammation of the bladder.

D & C: Dilatation and curettage. Spreading open (dilating) the cervix and scraping the inside of the uterus. In birthing, one need for this would be to clear away remaining pieces of the placenta.

Demerol: Proprietary name for meperidine or pethidine; an analgesic. Synthetic morphine.

Diabetes: A problem with sugar metabolism.

Diastasis: Separation of the abdominal muscles during pregnancy.

Dilation: Synonymous with dilatation. The expanding of the cervix (to ten centimeters) to allow the baby to pass through.

Diuretic: A substance used to stimulate urination.

Down's syndrome: Formerly called mongolism. A congenital condition, more common in babies born to mothers over forty (2.5 percent), characterized by mental and physical retardation.

Dyspnea: Difficult breathing.

Dystocia: Difficult labor. Shoulder dystocia comes about when one of the shoulders is blocked and trapped by the pelvic bone.

Eclampsia: Serious toxemia, indicated by high blood pressure, severe edema, convulsions, possible coma, and death if left untreated. Indicated by protein in the urine.

Ectopic pregnancy: A pregnancy in which the fertilized egg implants somewhere other than the walls of the uterus. The most common is when implantation takes place in the fallopian tube (tubal).

Edema: Swelling in various parts of the body, caused by retention of fluids. If generalized (body-wide), it is called dropsy. Localized edema, such as in the ankles, is common in the last months of pregnancy. Severe edema can be an indication of eclampsia or preeclampsia.

Effacement: Softening and thinning of the cervix, which allows dilation to occur. Usually expressed as a percentage.

Embryo: The new being, generally called an embryo up to the tenth week, after which it is called, in humans, a fetus.

Enema: A washing out of the rectum, both to be sure that a bowel movement during labor doesn't contaminate the birthing area and to stimulate contractions.

Engagement: When the presenting part of the baby (usually the head) moves into the pelvis.

Engorgement: When milk fills, or overfills, the breasts.

Epidural: A method of regional anesthesia in which the anesthetic is injected into the space just above the dura (outer membrane covering) of the spine. Often called an epidural block.

Episiotomy: A relatively minor surgical procedure in which a cut is made between the bottom of the vagina and across the perineum. The purpose is to create a larger opening to the birth canal, and thus prevent possible tearing.

Ergot: One of the primary parts of many oxytocics. Derived from a fungus that grows on various kinds of rye.

Estriol: A substance in the blood and urine of the mother. If the level of estriol falls, this is an indication of some kind of malfunction with the placenta.

Estrogens: A type of hormone. During pregnancy large quantities are secreted by the placenta, which cause the uterus, breasts, and external genitalia to enlarge and the glandular tissues in the breasts to grow. Estrogens also cause the pelvic ligaments to relax, allowing the pubic region to become more elastic.

Expulsion: When the baby comes out.

Fallopian tubes: The two "arms" that project from the sides of the uterus and deliver the egg from the ovaries to the uterus. Also called *oviducts*.

Fetal alcohol syndrome: A condition resulting from maternal alcohol consumption during pregnancy, which can include deformities, growth problems, and mental retardation.

Fetus: The unborn child. Generally considered to be after the tenth week or the third month of pregnancy. Before this it is commonly called an embryo.

FHR: Fetal heart rate.

FHT: Fetal heart tones.

First Stage: The period between the onset of labor and full cervical dilation.

Fontanel (or fontanelle): Soft spots on a baby's skull. These allow the skull to mold to the birth canal

Forceps: Tonglike instruments to assist in a difficult delivery.

Fundus: The upper part of the uterus.

GC: Test for gonorrhea.

Genitalia: The organs of reproduction, both internal and external.

Gestation: Period of pregnancy—how long it takes for the fetus to grow to term. In a human this is considered to be 280 days or 40 weeks.

Gestational diabetes: A common complication of pregnancy, detected by glucose tolerance tests.

Gluteus maximus: The primary muscles of the buttocks.

Gravid: Pregnant.

GTT: Glucose-tolerance test. Used to test for diabetes and hypoglycemia.

Gynecology: Medical study of women, particularly the reproductive organs.

HCT: Hemocrit, or a hemocrit blood test.

HGB: Hemoglobin, or a blood test for hemoglobin.

Hemocrit: The percentage of red blood cells as compared to the total quantity of blood. Also *hematocrit*.

Hemodilution: A natural increase in blood volume accompanied by a decrease in red blood cells. Occurs between twenty-eight and thirty-two weeks.

Hemorrhage: Excessive, and sometimes uncontrollable, bleeding.

HPL: Human placental lactogen. A hormone found in higher concentrations in pregnant women, with the level rising up to about thirty-six weeks.

Human chorionic gonadotropin: A substance found in the urine of pregnant women a few days after implantation and which reaches a peak about sixty days after the last period.

Hydramnios: An overly abundant amount of amniotic fluid.

Hydrocephalus: Enlarged cranium.

Hymen: A thin membrane that partially covers the vaginal opening. Usually breaks upon first intercourse, if not before. In a few cases it remains intact, or partially intact, until the birth of a child.

Hyperemesis gravidarum: Serious morning sickness.

Hypertension: High blood pressure.

Hyperventilation: When the amount of carbon dioxide in the blood is depleted, such as through rapid breathing. Characterized by dizziness and possible fainting.

Hypotension: Low blood pressure.

Hypoxia: When the fetus is not getting sufficient oxygen while in the uterus, such as when the cord is compressed or if the placenta breaks loose too soon (abruptio placentae). Causes fetal distress and may become an emergency situation.

Hysterectomy: Removal of the uterus by surgery.

Implantation: When the fertilized ovum (egg) moves down the fallopian tube, into the uterus, and embeds itself in the endometrium. This usually takes place on the seventh or eighth day after ovulation.

Induction: Stimulation of labor through artificial means, such as through the use of pitocin.

Inverted nipple: When the nipple is flat or depressed rather than jutting out. Can cause difficulty in nursing, but can usually be cured.

Involution: Reduction in size of the uterus after the birth, and a gradual return to a normal, nonpregnant state.

IUD: Intrauterine device. A method of contraception.

Jaundice: Yellowing, most often caused by breakdown of red blood cells with bilirubin as a byproduct. Very common in neonates. Can also be caused by Rh incompatibility, blood type incompatibility (ABO syndrome), infection, hormones in the breast milk, liver malfunction, or blocked ducts.

Kegel exercises: Named after Dr. Arnold H. Kegel. A set of exercises that help to tone and condition the PC muscle(s), consisting primarily of contracting and relaxing the muscles.

Labia: The "lips" of the female genitalia. The labia majora are the larger, fleshier outer lips, while the labia minora are the smaller inner ones.

Labor: The process of birthing, particularly the contractions and pushing.

Laceration: A tearing of tissues or muscles.

Lactation: Producing and secreting milk for breast-feeding.

La Leche League International: An organization concerned with the promotion of breast-feeding.

Lanugo: Fine hair covering the fetus.

LDR: Labor-delivery-recovery; a term sometimes used by hospitals or others to describe a single room that can be used for all three.

Letdown: The process of milk in the breasts moving from the alveoli and into the ducts. Stimulated by oxytocin.

Lightening: When the baby drops lower in the uterus just prior to birth (the last weeks of pregnancy). Pressure above is lessened, while pressure lower is increased, sometimes causing pains in the legs. Abdominal shape changes. Also called *dropping*.

Linea nigra: A dark line (pigmentation) that forms during many pregnancies from the pubic area to the navel (and sometimes beyond).

Lithotomy position: The most common birthing position used in hospitals; with the woman on her back with legs spread and in stirrups. This is easiest for the doctor, but not so great for the mother since she is pushing against gravity.

Lochia: Uterine discharges after the birth. During the first six days the discharge is blood-tinged (lochia rubra or lochia cruenta). The next three to four days it becomes brownish in appearance (lochia serosa). Finally it becomes yellowish and white (lochia alba).

L/S ratio: A test to determine the ratio of lecithin and sphingomyelin in the amniotic fluid, via amniocentesis. Common before induction of labor or cesarean births if either the mother or baby seem to be at risk. The test determines the maturity and development of the baby's lungs.

Malpresentation: A condition where the fetus is in an awkward or possibly dangerous position in the uterus.

Mammary: Having to do with the breasts.

"Mask of pregnancy": Darkening of parts of the body, usually the face. Marks can be red, purple, and sometimes brown.

Mastitis: Infection of the breast, particularly the milk ducts. Often caused by prolonged breast engorgement.

MCH: Mean corpuscular hemoglobin. A blood test to determine the amount of hemoglobin in the red blood cells.

MCHC: Mean corpuscular hemoglobin concentration. A blood test to determine the relative amount of hemoglobin per size of red blood cell.

MCV: Mean corpuscular volume. A blood test to determine the size of red blood cells.

Meconium: The first bowel movements of the baby. These are dark green to black and tarry in appearance.

Menses: "Month." Used to refer to the monthly menstrual cycle or sexual cycle of the female. Commonly called a "period."

Menopause: When the female is no longer able to bear children.

Midwife: Someone, not necessarily a doctor and almost always a woman, who assists in childbirth. C.N.M.s (certified nurse midwives) are registered nurses with extensive training in childbirth.

Monilia: Older and now rarely used name for Candida, a yeastlike fungus.

Montgomery's tubercles: Small bumps around the areola that increase in size during pregnancy.

Moro reflex: An automatic defensive response in the neonate in which its arms spread in a drop or close up tight if the baby's resting surface is slapped.

Mucus plug: A plug made up of mucus and blood that blocks the cervix during pregnancy and breaks loose just before the birth.

Nembutal: Trade name for pentobarbital. A barbiturate once used to cause sleep for mothers in labor. It was found to decrease fetal respiration to a dangerous degree.

Neonatal: Having to do with the newborn child (neonate).

Nesting instinct: The tendency of a pregnant woman to want to clean up the house just before labor begins. Characterized by high energy. Often Mom doesn't even realize that she is doing it.

Ob-gyn: Obstetrics gynecology. Combined medical studies concerning the female reproductive systems, pregnancy, and birthing.

Obstetrics: The medical study and practice of pregnancy and birth. The origin of the word is Latin, and means "midwife."

Occiput: The back of the skull.

OCT: Oxytocin challenge test. Used to stimulate temporary contractions.

Os: An opening. Particularly in birthing, the opening of the cervix in the uterus.

Ovum: The egg. Comes from the ovary in a process called ovulation.

Oxytocin: A hormone. Sometimes used to stimulate (induce) labor. Occurs naturally during breast-feeding, thus speeding the process of involution (return to normal), or during breast massage to help stimulate contractions. From the pituitary gland. Synthetic oxytocin is pitocin. Oxytocics are a variety of labor-stimulating substances.

Palpation: Exploration by feel.

Pap smear: Short for Papanicolaou after the scientist who developed the test. A light scraping of the tissues, particularly of the vagina and cervix, in order to test for cancer and other abnormal changes in the cells.

Paracervical block: Local anesthetic injected between the cervix and vagina. Not often used in modern medicine due to depression of fetal and neonatal respiration and heartbeat.

Parity: The number of pregnancies the woman has had.

Parturition: The process of birth. The parturient is the woman in labor.

PC muscle(s): Pubococcygeus muscle(s), sometimes called the Kegel muscle(s). Five muscles that hold the uterus, bladder, lower bowel, and vagina. Closely associated with the sphincter muscles of the vagina and anus.

Pediatrics: The branch of medicine related to the treatment of children.

Pelvic: Having to do with the pelvis or the region of the pelvis. The first physical examination and those of the last weeks of pregnancy might be "pelvic" exams, which means that the physician visually and manually examines the genitals and reproductive tract of the woman.

Pelvic floor: The perineum. Located between the vagina and

the anus. Cutting the muscles of this area is an episiotomy.

Pelvis: Often thought of as the hip bones. More accurately it is the "trough" (Greek translation of *pyelos*, from which we get pelvis) between the hip bones and the spine.

Perinatal: The period just before, during, and particularly just after the birth.

Perinatology: Care of the newborn.

Perineum: Floor of the pelvis. Located between the bottom of the vagina and the anus.

Pitting: Depressions that remain after pushing against an area swollen by edema.

Pitocin: Proprietary name for synthetic oxytocin. Sometimes called Pit.

PKU Test: A neonatal blood test required by most states to test for a condition called phenylketonuria. This is an inability, to some degree, of the baby's digestive system to handle the amino acid phenylalanine. This condition can cause serious mental retardation but is easily treated.

Placenta: An organ that forms during pregnancy and which is attached to the uterus on one side and through the umbilical cord to the fetus on the other. Allows passage of blood between mother and fetus, thus providing the fetus with oxygen and nourishment (and sometimes undesirable substances), while removing wastes from the body of the fetus. Weighs about one pound. Delivery of the placenta is called the *afterbirth*.

Placenta accreta: A condition in which the placenta becomes attached to the uterine muscle, making release extremely difficult, and often requiring surgery.

Placenta previa: When the placenta forms over or near the cervix. Indicated by painless bleeding during the last few months of pregnancy. If complete (placenta previa centralis) or partial (placenta previa marginalis), the placenta is blocking the cervix, and cesarean section is required.

Placental souffle: Sound made by circulation of blood, and heard over the placenta. A blowing sound.

Plateau phenomenon: A pausing in labor, usually when the cervix has dilated to four centimeters, again at seven centimeters and again at nine centimeters.

Pneumonia: An inflammation in the lungs. If the fetus breathes in (aspirates) fluids or meconium during birth, or suffers an infection, pneumonia can result.

Polyhydramnios: Excessive amniotic fluid. Caused by multiple pregnancy (twins, etc.), toxemia, diabetes, or various fetal anomalies. Also called *hydramnios*.

Posterior: Back or toward the rear. Posterior presentation is when the baby is facing the wrong direction during birth, often causing back labor.

Postpartum: After the birth.

Postpartum depression: Depression of the mother following the birth, experienced by up to 80 percent of all women.

Precutaneous umbilical blood sampling: A test to detect chromosomal abnormalities. A needle is inserted into the umbilical cord to get a sample of blood.

Preeclampsia: A form of toxemia, and a less severe form of eclampsia.

Premature: A birth in which the child is of thirty-six weeks of gestation or less, and/or has a body weight of five and one half pounds or less. Sometimes called a preemie.

Prep: Preparing the mother for the birth. Particularly concerning the pubic shave.

Prepuce: The covering of the clitoris.

Presentation: How the fetus is coming out.

Primigravida: First pregnancy; with *primi* meaning first and *gravida* being a term for pregnancy.
(*Multigravida* would mean someone who is having a second, third, or whatever child.) Also called *primipara*.

Progesterone: A hormone secreted by the ovaries and by the

placenta during pregnancy. Decreases uterine contractions, and thus prevents spontaneous abortion. Also helps to prepare the breasts for lactation.

Prolactin: A hormone secreted by the anterior pituitary gland that works with other hormones, particularly estrogen and progesterone, to prepare the breasts and to stimulate lactation.

Prolapse: When the umbilical cord drops into the birth canal ahead of the baby. Almost always necessitates a cesarean section.

Proteinuria: Protein in the urine, indicating possible eclampsia.

Pseudocyesis: False pregnancy.

Pudendum: The external genitalia of a female. A pudendal block is a regional anesthetic given in this area, administered in late labor and for an episiotomy and repair of the same.

Puerperal: Having to do with birth. Puerperal fever, more correctly called puerperal sepsis or puerperal septicemia, also called childbed fever, is caused by an infection of the birth tract.

Puerperium: The six weeks after the birth of the child.

RDS: Respiratory distress syndrome. Caused by underdeveloped lungs. More common in premature babies. Sometimes called hyaline membrane disease.

Rh: A factor in the blood, either + (positive) or − (negative), with Rh+ being the most common, indicating certain antibodies are present, and Rh− being an absence of those antibodies. Can be of concern if the mother is Rh− and the fetus Rh+, since this can cause the mother's body to produce possibly detrimental antibodies. These can harm the baby and any future babies she might have.

RhoGAM: An antiantigen given to Rh− mothers immediately after birth to prevent problems then and in future births.

Rooting reflex: An automatic response in a child to turn toward and start sucking at something that touches its cheek.

Rubella: German measles. Very dangerous for the fetus.

Saddle block: A type of regional anesthesia given in the fourth lumbar (lower spine) that desensitizes the perineum and buttocks—where the body would touch a saddle. Also called a "little spinal."

Sciatica: Shooting pains in the legs. Caused by the fetus pressing on the sciatic nerve in the spine.

Scopolamine: A drug of the hallucinogenic/amnesic variety. Causes what is known as "twilight sleep." The mother feels the pain of birth, but forgets it.

Second stage: The period between when the cervix is fully dilated and the birth of the child.

Sepsis: Infection.

Sickle-cell anemia: A hereditary disease specific to African-Americans in which the red blood cells have a crescent shape and contain hemoglobin S.

SIDS: Sudden infant death syndrome. Also called crib death. There is no known cause or cure. Sometimes an apnea alarm mattress is used, which signals when breathing stops.

Sinciput: The forehead, or bones of the forehead.

Sonogram: Sound used to create a picture of the baby in the womb and to diagnose certain problems, such as twins, placenta previa, etc. See also *ultrasound*.

Souffle: A blowing sound, such as with uterine souffle.

Spina bifida: Exposed spinal meninges. Potentially fatal. Also called spinal bifida.

Station: Position of the fetus in relation to the pelvis just before birth. Indicated as positive or negative numbers, with −4 being high, 0 being engagement, and +4 being crowning.

Striae: Stretch marks, generally white and shiny, such as on the abdomen after birth or on the breasts after weaning. Specifically, striae gravidarum are stretch marks during or caused by pregnancy.

Succenturiata: Placental succenturiata is when there is a separate lobe to the placenta, which often stays behind in the uterus and can cause heavy bleeding. The indication is if a piece of the placenta is missing and blood vessels on the fetal side come to a stop.

Suture: A joint. Can be a joint between bones, or a man-made joint of tissues by sewing. Sometimes used to describe the thread used to make the stitch.

Symphysis pubis: The joint of the pubic bones in the center and front of the pubic area and just beneath the pubic hair.

Tachycardia: Rapid heart rate.

Tay-Sachs disease: A hereditary disease specific to Jewish parents. Almost always fatal within eighteen months of birth. Amniocentesis is done to test for the enzyme hexosamidase A. If this enzyme is present in either parent, the child will not contract the disease.

Term: Full duration of pregnancy (280 days) and when birth takes place.

Third stage: The period after the birth of the child and delivery of the placenta. Normally between thirty and forty-five minutes of the birth.

Thrush: A common disease in newborns characterized by small white patches and/or ulcers, particularly in the mouth and throat. Often caused by a vaginal yeast infection from the mother.

Toxemia: A form of blood poisoning that occurs during pregnancy, and characterized by edema, hypertension, fever, and possible vomiting, among other symptoms. See also eclampsia and preeclampsia.

Toxoplasmosis: A disease spread by uncooked meat and fish, birds (their feces), and cats (their feces). Dangerous for the fetus, and very likely one of the main reasons why you might hear that you should get rid of your cat if Mom is pregnant.

Transition: When the cervix is between eight and ten centimeters in dilation and the baby's head is passing through the cervix and into the birth canal.

Transverse: Sideways. Describes position of the fetus. A transverse position is normal up to about twenty-six weeks. It can cause serious problems.

Trichomonas: A vaginal infection caused by a parasitic protozoa. Can move into the bladder. Characterized by itching and burning and a frothy white discharge. Sometimes called "trich." See also Candida.

Trimester: One of the three periods of pregnancy. For example, the first three months are the first trimester, while the last three months are the third trimester.

Ultrasound: A technique used to "look" inside the womb using sound instead of X rays. New evidence shows a concern that it *might* be potentially dangerous. See *sonogram*.

Umbilical cord: The cord that connects the fetus to the mother through the placenta.

Umbilicus: The belly button.

Urethra: The opening through which urine leaves the body.

Uterus: A musclar organ in which the fetus develops. The womb.

Vacuum extraction: An alternative to forceps delivery, in which suction is used instead of mechanical forceps.

Vagina: The birth canal. A muscular and sheathlike organ between the cervix and the external genitalia.

VDRL: More correctly called VDRL-STS, for Venereal Disease Research Laboratory—Serological Test for Syphilis.

Vernix: A protective skinlike covering over the fetus while it is in the uterus.

Vertex: The top of the head or skull. A vertex presentation

would be a birth in which the top of the head comes first.

Vulva: The female's external genitalia. Also called the *pudendum*.

Water: In birthing, refers to the amniotic fluid.

Index